Health Essentials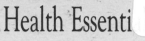

Acupuncture

Peter Mole studied Modern History at Oxford University before training to be an an acupuncturist. He now practises at the Oxford Acupuncture Centre and teaches at the College of Traditional Acupuncture. He is currently the President of the Traditional Acupuncture Society.

The Health Essentials Series

There is a growing number of people who find themselves attracted to holistic or alternative therapies and natural approaches to maintaining optimum health and vitality. The *Health Essentials* series is designed to help the newcomer by presenting high quality introductions to all the main complementary health subjects. Each book presents all the essential information on each therapy, explaining what it is, how it works and what it can do for the reader. Advice is also given, where possible, on how to begin using the therapy at home, together with comprehensive lists of courses and classes available worldwide.

The *Health Essentials* titles are all written by practising experts in their fields. Exceptionally clear and concise, each text is supported by attractive illustrations.

Series Medical Consultant
Dr John Cosh MD, FRCP

In the same series

Alexander Technique by Richard Brennan
Aromatherapy by Christine Wildwood
Flower Remedies by Christine Wildwood
Reflexology by Inge Dougans with Suzanne Ellis
Shiatsu by Elaine Liechti
Skin and Body Care by Sidra Shaukat
Spiritual Healing by Jack Angelo

Health Essentials

ACUPUNCTURE

Energy Balancing for Body, Mind and Spirit

PETER MOLE
BA, MAc, MTAB

ELEMENT
Shaftesbury, Dorset ● Rockport, Massachusetts
Brisbane, Queensland

© Peter Mole 1992

Published in Great Britain in 1992 by
Element Books Limited
Longmead, Shaftesbury, Dorset

Published in the USA in 1992 by
Element, Inc
42 Broadway, Rockport, MA 01966

Published in Australia by
Element Books Ltd for
Jacaranda Wiley Ltd
33 Park Road, Milton, Brisbane, 4064

Cover illustration from an Eric Gill woodcut
Cover design by Max Fairbrother
Typeset by Falcon Typographic Art Ltd, Fife, Scotland
Printed and bound in Great Britain by
Billings Ltd, Hylton Road, Worcester

A catalogue record for this book
is available from the British Library

Library of Congress Cataloging-in-Publication Data

Mole, Peter.
Acupuncture : energy balancing for body, mind, and spirit
Peter Mole.
Includes bibliographical references and index.
1. Acupuncture.   I. Title.   II. Series: Health essentials series.
RM184.M62   1992   615.8'92 – dc20   92–6137

ISBN 1–85230–319–0

Note from the Publisher

Any information given in any book in the *Health Essentials* series is not intended to be taken as a replacement for medical advice. Any person with a condition requiring medical attention should consult a qualified medical practitioner or suitable therapist.

Contents

Author's Note

THIS BOOK IS intended to be a source of information on the subject of acupuncture to patients, prospective patients, prospective students and lay-people in general. It is *not* intended to be a sort of 'home doctor' which the reader can consult in order to make an acupuncture diagnosis of his own or others' symptoms. One of the intentions of the book is to show that acupuncture has a complex and intricate diagnostic method which takes a practitioner many years in which to become adept. If the book serves to show that acupuncture offers a radically different approach from Western medicine and that symptoms can rarely be seen out of context of the person as a whole, then it will have gone some way to fulfilling its purpose.

I decided to resolve the problem of whether to use the masculine or feminine pronoun throughout the book by using them alternately in each chapter. Unfortunately the book has seven chapters and, decided by the toss of a coin, this has meant that the masculine pronoun has been used in one more chapter than the feminine.

I would like to thank all the people who by their lectures, books, friendship and example have contributed to my education in the art and science of acupuncture. In particular my first teacher J. R. Worsley, whose inspiring use of acupuncture to treat the person's mind and spirit has profoundly influenced me; Allegra Wint, my companion and fellow-acupuncturist since my early days in practice; Angie and John Hicks, Ted Kaptchuk, Giovanni Maciocia, Claude Larre and Elizabeth Rochat de La Vallée.

I would also like to thank all the people who have been kind enough to read sections of this book and, by their comments and suggestions, have helped to clarify my thinking and writing: Margaret Mole, Ken Shifrin, Amanda Thurston, Alan Hext and Freda Wint. Special thanks to Pat Utechin for the index.

Finally I would like to dedicate this book to my three children: Guy, Toby and Jessica, in the hope that when they are older they will gain some understanding of the nature of their father's work and why he stopped playing with them sometimes.

1

What Is Traditional Acupuncture? How Is It Different From Western Medicine?

I N THE 1970S it was quite usual to meet people who had never heard of acupuncture. Media coverage in recent years has ensured that almost everybody has at least heard of it and is aware that it originated in China, that it involves inserting needles into the patient and that it is extremely effective. Beyond that, very little is commonly known about this elegant and sophisticated system of medicine.

Acupuncture is one of the principal components – along with herbalism, massage and other therapies – of an age-old

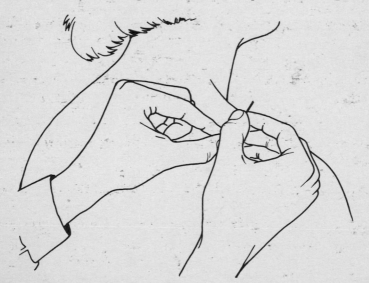

Fig. 1. Acupuncture treatment

system of medicine known as Chinese medicine.[1] This is one of the very few traditional medical systems which continues to hold its own in the face of the dominance of the Western medical model. Based on ancient texts, it has been the subject of continuous study, assessment and clinical experience over thousands of years, treating billions of patients.

Any person who professes to practise acupuncture without having studied Chinese medical theory and who maintains that it can be used as an adjunct to Western medicine[2] has failed to grasp its essence. It is hard to know whether to laugh or cry over the recent trend of doctors to set themselves up as acupuncturists after courses lasting only two week-ends.[3] It is analogous to a lay-person practising surgery without having studied anatomy and physiology.

Traditional acupuncture, hitherto practised extensively throughout the Orient, is now growing rapidly in popularity throughout the rest of the world. It is based on a detailed and subtle diagnosis of an individual's particular needs. No two patients are ever treated identically even if, to the untrained observer, their symptoms appear virtually identical. When Western medicine first came to the East, the traditional physicians were amazed that the doctors gave exactly the same remedies to all their patients suffering from the same symptoms without making any attempt to diagnose each individual's constitutional weaknesses or even the cause of the complaint. Chuang Tse (4th century BC), a leading Daoist thinker wrote:

> Natures differ, and needs with them,
> Hence the wise men of old
> did not lay down
> One measure for all.

A HOLISTIC THERAPY

In a medical context, the word 'holistic' (from the Greek word *holos* meaning whole) means treating the patient *as a whole*, rather than treating the symptoms out of context of the human being who has the symptoms. Sickness is not understood in terms of the pathology of isolated organs, as though they were merely cogs in a machine, but rather as the dysfunction of a normally harmonious, complete living entity.

Chinese medicine never considered the mind and body as separate from each other, as Western medicine has for the last two centuries. This may sound like a cliché, but it gives the two systems a fundamentally different philosophical basis which permeates to the core of their theories and practice. The belief that the human body is little more than an extremely sophisticated machine has led, in the West, to many extraordinary advances; for example, the remarkable developments in surgery and drug therapy. Much of the current disaffection with modern medicine amongst patients, however, stems from the limitations of this approach. It fails to recognize that the mind and spirit have an extremely powerful effect upon the body and that the human body is more than the sum of its chemistry and mechanics.

All systems of medicine can be practised more or less holistically, depending on the wisdom of the physician. What is remarkable about Chinese medicine is that it places diagnosis of the *person* at the core of its diagnostic process and regards nearly all chronic disease as a manifestation of that individual's particular weaknesses. When acupuncture treatment is directed at these long-standing weaknesses or 'imbalances', the patient is often amazed to find that not only is his main complaint improving, but many secondary complaints are also responding. This contrasts significantly with the effect of many of the modern drugs which, because of their side-effects, create secondary complaints rather than improve them.

This improvement in the patient's well-being as a whole is one of the main reasons that patients in the West have been flocking to acupuncturists over the last few decades. Their holistic acupuncture treatment is in marked contrast to the treatment they receive from the gamut of specialists they are accustomed to seeing, as they trawl round the various out-patient departments of our hospitals. It is indicative of the nature of acupuncture that none of its leading colleges grant qualifications in any speciality. Acupuncturists have always specialized in treating human beings, not illnesses.

What an acupuncturist is searching for when he sees a patient are the 'patterns of disharmony' which have caused the symptoms now afflicting the patient. For example, if a Western doctor and an acupuncturist were both to examine a patient with difficulty in breathing, the doctor might diagnose asthma and the acupuncturist might diagnose a deficiency in the 'energy' of the lung. It is not that one is correct and the other incorrect; it is just that they both see the symptom through the perception of their own very different medical models.

Acupuncture has recently become famous for its ability to treat pain, but historically it has always been used to treat the entire spectrum of disease. A patient may come to the acupuncturist with any symptom at all, whether primarily psychological in expression, for example, depression or anxiety, or any one of the huge number of possible physical complaints. The acupuncturist's response is always the same – to diagnose the pattern of disharmony of that unique individual before deciding on the relevant treatment.

People often ask if acupuncture is appropriate for this symptom or that symptom and the answer is essentially always the same: if the practitioner is able to make an accurate diagnosis of the pattern of disharmony, then acupuncture will improve the healthy functioning, the 'well-being', of the patient's body, mind and spirit. Sometimes this means that the symptoms will be completely cured and sometimes the disease process has advanced too far for that to be possible. In these cases acupuncture can enhance the person's state of health to the extent that the symptoms are diminished in intensity, frequency and duration.

People also often ask if acupuncture can help in so-called 'incurable' disease. There are many recorded instances of people recovering from 'incurable' illnesses, whether through the medium of acupuncture, Western medicine, prayer or many other forms of healing. Usually, however, the acupuncturist can only improve the quality of life for the patient, physically, mentally and spiritually. As the poet John Milton observed: 'It is not miserable to be blind; it is miserable to be incapable of enduring blindness'.

The great physician, Sir William Osler (1849–1919), said 'Don't tell me what type of disease the patient has, tell me what type of patient has the disease'. In the case of a chronic symptom, the acupuncturist would agree with that view. Treatment is primarily focused on the deep-seated *cause* of a chronic illness. In acute conditions, the acupuncturist may first concentrate on the symptoms and treat the underlying weakness secondarily.

People by the roadside in many Third World countries beg for aspirin; for them it is a wonder drug. It is, for example, in many ways an excellent remedy for the acute condition of having a headache. What it does not treat, however, is the chronic condition of having headaches. While one is extremely grateful for symptomatic relief, such as that provided by the aspirin, one of the fundamental axioms of acupuncture, is: 'a disease that is not completely cured can easily breed new disease or there can be a relapse of the old disease'. Western medicine is now very popular with patients throughout the East for its efficacy in treating acute symptoms but often they will use traditional medicine to treat their chronic symptoms. It is in the treatment of long-standing chronic disease that acupuncture has most to offer the patient in the West. As it says in the *Nei Jing* (2nd century BC: the principal Classic of Chinese medicine), 'Even if a disease is of long duration it can be cured; those who say it cannot be cured do not know acupuncture properly'.

It must be said that there are obviously situations where it is not appropriate to treat holistically, for example in emergencies or for symptoms caused by physical injury. If I were to be in a serious car crash then I would have no wish to be taken in the first instance to an acupuncturist. Although there is a long tradition of using acupuncture as first-aid, there is no doubt that in cases of serious physical injury Western medicine is the preferred therapy. After the emergency has been dealt with, however, acupuncture is extremely valuable for its ability to help the person to recover from the effect of the shock and trauma.

THE PRINCIPLES OF RESTORING HEALTH THROUGH ACUPUNCTURE

Human beings have extraordinary powers of recovery; if they did not then each fever, each emotional trauma, each stress or injury would leave the person a physical or emotional wreck. The natural disposition of the body, mind and spirit to gravitate back towards a state of equilibrium is known as homoeostasis. The aim of the acupuncturist is to assist these homoeostatic functions. The elimination of symptoms may often be an important immediate goal of treatment but it is not its fundamental or ultimate goal.

It is common for patients to report after a number of treatments that they now feel as they used to before a certain event or period of their life which undermined their health. Many people have a sense of themselves in which they know that they are not achieving their full potential in terms of physical, mental or spiritual vitality. It is essential that the practitioner has a clear sense of how the patient *could* be when he is restored to a state of health – to recognize what is an appropriate level of vitality and health, bearing in mind the individual's age, constitution and circumstances.

The principle of the doctor striving to restore healthy function rather than endeavouring to 'fight' illness is an old-established, if currently unfashionable, one in Western medicine. It seems to have particularly died out in the English-speaking medical profession. It still, however, holds a great deal of sway in Europe. In France the concept of strengthening the individual's *terrain*, or underlying state of health, is still very much in vogue. In Germany, for example, antibiotics are prescribed approximately half as often as they are in the UK, where doctors prescribe them considerably less often than their counterparts in the USA. Dr Peter Naumann, Professor of infectious diseases at the University of Dusseldorf, says 'There are no real indications for giving antibiotics in private practice. If a patient needs an antibiotic, he generally needs to be in hospital.' This contrast with current prescribing habits in the UK and USA could hardly have been put more starkly.

The fundamental difference is that German doctors still concentrate much of their treatment on enhancing the patient's own powers of recovery. Hydrotherapy, in various forms, is commonly prescribed by doctors to help the patient throw off an infection and this is funded by all the German health insurance schemes. About one-fifth of German doctors practise either homoeopathic, anthroposophic or herbal medicine. These, as well as vitamin therapy, are frequently used to help restore health.

An interesting example of acupuncture being used to promote health rather than to 'fight' illness is in the treatment of AIDS. In the USA and UK especially, thousands of HIV-positive and AIDS patients have reported great improvements in their overall health and well-being, due to their 'health-promoting' treatment by traditional acupuncture. At the time of writing it is still too early to say exactly how effective the treatment is, but until or unless Western medicine develops greatly improved treatments acupuncture will remain one of the principal therapies of choice for sufferers from these syndromes.

A FORM OF PREVENTIVE MEDICINE

The ability of acupuncture to promote healthy functioning means that it is often used as an effective form of *preventive medicine*. Preventive medicine in the West is predominantly limited by the fact that, even when a diagnostic test does discern dysfunction before symptoms have arisen, treatment is usually limited to the reduction of illness-producing factors such as poor diet, lack of exercise or excessive stress. Virtually nothing can ever be done to improve the function of the ailing organ or system itself. A famous passage in the *Nei Jing* states one of the fundamental axioms of acupuncture:

> When medicinal therapy is initiated only after someone has fallen ill, when there is an attempt to restore order only after unrest has broken out, it is as though someone has waited to dig a well until he is already weak from thirst, or as if someone begins to forge a spear when the battle is already underway. Is this not too late?

It is obvious that serious organic diseases, such as cardiac failure, diabetes or cancer do not arise overnight. They are always preceded by a breakdown in healthy function which has eventually led to the disease reaching the organic stage. This, in the opinion of acupuncturists, represents an advanced stage of a disease. This is also true for the majority of less severe, but chronic, illnesses from which most people suffer. A skilful acupuncturist, using traditional methods of diagnosis, can often detect and treat disorders in an individual's healthy functioning long before they develop into symptoms discernible either to the person or to the diagnostic procedures of Western medicine. In the early years of acupuncture in the West, nearly all the patients who were prepared to try this unfamiliar therapy were already suffering from the advanced stages of their illnesses and were coming to acupuncture as a last resort. Many people in recent years however, having heard of acupuncture's use as preventive medicine, have been consulting acupuncture practitioners at much earlier stages in the disease process. This enables them to maintain and improve their level of health, rather than beginning 'to forge a spear when the battle is already underway'.

Not only does the use of acupuncture help to prevent the onset of illnesses induced by the person's own energetic imbalances, but it also enhances the person's resistance to infectious disease. Western medicine has no satisfactory explanation for why, given that we are constantly exposed to bacteria and viruses, our immune systems are intermittently ineffective. The Chinese view is that the occurrence of disease from infection is due to the struggle between the infective agent and the person's 'energy' or 'vital-force'. If the individual's state of health is excellent then it is very difficult for an infection to overcome the body's natural defences. It is true, however, that Chinese medicine was never very effective against the appalling epidemics that ravaged China, and the rest of the East, until modern times. It is an extraordinary irony that these countries, which developed such a refined system of internal medicine, had never managed to ensure such essential public health measures as clean water or efficient waste disposal. For many patients in the West, however, no longer prey to typhoid, cholera and bubonic plague, acupuncture has been extremely successful in helping to build up their resistance to such infections as cystitis, bronchitis, pneumonia, colds, and such like.

WHAT IS AN ACUPUNCTURIST'S VIEW OF HEALTH?

It is quite common for an individual to go for a medical check-up and, after a number of investigations, to be told that they are in 'perfect shape' or 'A.1'. For the traditional acupuncturist there is no real concept of 'perfect health'. Perhaps the closest a human being ever comes to that state is as a very young baby, but even here there are probably already slight imbalances which are either inherited, acquired in the womb or due to birth trauma. For the rest of us too much water has flowed under the bridge in the form of illness, trauma and stress, for there not to be imbalances discernible to the acupuncturist. The health of the individual depends on the severity of the imbalances: we are all unhealthy, it is a purely a question of degree. Fortunately for many people this does not necessarily mean that they have physical symptoms that ail them. To the acupuncturist, however, health is not judged by physical health alone. Assessment of the person's spirit, mind and emotions are of prime importance.

The *Huainanzi* (2nd century BC), one of the Classics of ancient Chinese scientific thought, put it like this:

> What is it that gives man clear vision and fine hearing, a straight body whose parts flex and stretch easily? What allows him to distinguish black and white through observation, beautiful and ugly through consideration, and, through appreciation, the similar and the different, the things that are appropriate and those that are not? It is the abundance of the energy and the activity of the spirit.

For the Chinese, their legendary quest for longevity was not a search for an inordinate extension of their life-span. As the sinologist Claude Larre states, it was, 'the pursuit of the perfect working of a being who, according to his nature, completes the measure of his destiny and dies in his own time'.

WHAT IS QI?

The concept of Qi (formerly spelt ch'i, pronounced chee) lies at the very heart of acupuncture. For those of us who have been brought up in the West, taking on board the notion of Qi is the conceptual leap that we have to make in order to understand Chinese medicine.[4]

Unless one can accept the validity of the existence of Qi, then acupuncture, not to mention Tai Ji Quan, the oriental martial arts, Yoga and many other Eastern practices, will remain a mystery. For people who have grown up in the East, the concept of Qi forms an integral part of their view of the human being. In different countries it has different names and is perceived slightly differently. In Japan it is called Ki; in India it is known as Prana; in Tibet, Rlun.

What the peoples of all these countries are referring to is the idea that living matter contains 'energy'. Many people have tried to translate Qi in other ways that more literally describe what it means to the Chinese. 'Life force', 'Vital force', 'Matter-energy', 'Breaths' and many other expressions, have been put forward by different translators to attempt to convey into English a concept that barely exists in our thought and culture. Qi is simply that which makes us alive. At our death it leaves us to return to the 'Great Void'. Wang Chong (AD 27–97) said:

> Qi produces the human body just as water becomes ice. As water freezes into ice, so Qi coagulates to form the human body. When ice melts, it becomes water. When a person dies, he or she becomes spirit again. It is called spirit, just as melted ice changes its name to water.

Chinese medicine is founded upon the study and observation of Qi: its flow, rhythms, cycles, changes, movement and balance. All traditional acupuncturists strive to deepen their understanding of the nature of the patient's Qi in order to determine how best they can use their skill to bring him back to a more harmonious state of health.

Chinese medicine places great emphasis on the relationship between human beings and their environment. Profound changes take place in our Qi with changes in the weather and the cycle of the seasons. Qi is not only present in all living matter but is present throughout the universe. In the *Nei Jing* it says 'The union of the Heaven and the Earth is called the human being'. This idea is reflected daily in our lives through our constant physical need to replenish our Qi from the air that we breathe and the food that we eat. This, combined with the Qi we inherit from our parents, forms the basis of our energetic constitution. Illness is seen as a dysfunction of Qi and acupuncture is a time-honoured method of regulating and enhancing a person's energetic system.

For example, a patient may complain to his doctor of lethargy and the conscientious physician will attempt to ascertain if there is any pathology, for example, glandular fever, anaemia, etc. There is, however, very often no discernible pathological cause and the patient is probably sent away without treatment or possibly diagnosed as suffering from depression. (In France, Germany and other countries in Europe he would probably be offered vitamins, a tonic or a visit to one of the many thriving spas.) To the acupuncturist, the patient is suffering from a dysfunction of his Qi and he will seek to diagnose and treat the energetic cause of the patient's lethargy.

All therapeutic interventions from any system of medicine indirectly affect a patient's Qi; one of acupuncture's strengths is its ability to affect an individual's Qi directly and powerfully. Only when the acupuncturist has completed his diagnosis and has reached a firm conclusion as to the condition of the patient's energetic balance, will he consider making a therapeutic intervention in the Qi of the patient. Any person who uses acupuncture and treats without having made a diagnosis of that particular person's energetic imbalances (except in the case of emergency first-aid) has violated one of the fundamental principles of Chinese medicine.

This, regrettably, is becoming more common in the West as some people try to practise this intricate system of medicine without even studying its basic principles, let alone its subtleties. For the first time in history, modern technology has developed machines, now on sale to the general public, that have made the job of the incompetent considerably easier. By detecting areas of high electrical conductivity relative to nearby tissues, these machines reveal where the acupuncture points are. The accompanying leaflet tells the customer how to use the same machine to treat particular points for particular symptoms, according to a Western medical model of symptoms. One can hardly be surprised if the therapeutic results are less than impressive. One suspects that the ancient Chinese practitioners must be whirling in their graves.

HOW DOES AN ACUPUNCTURIST TREAT SOMEONE'S QI?

> The means whereby man is created, the means whereby disease occurs, the means whereby man is cured, whereby disease arises: the twelve meridians are the basis of all theory and treatment.
>
> *Nei Jing*

The crucial breakthrough that enabled the Chinese to develop the practice of acupuncture was the discovery of 'points' on the body at which they could affect the Qi of the individual. This happened at least three thousand years ago and archaeological evidence suggests that it may have been considerably earlier. The belief that acupuncture was discovered by soldiers noticing that their symtoms improved when they were wounded in various spots (a view seemingly commonly held amongst newspaper cartoonists) has never been taken seriously by acupuncturists. Many of the points are tender on palpation and it is probable that most were discovered by early physicians exploring their patients' bodies for painful sites.[5] The other way in which the points, and the pathways between them, may have been discovered is through certain adepts focusing their attention during meditation on extremely subtle sensations in their bodies, much as some Indians did when they discovered the chakras of Hatha Yoga. Certainly many patients become aware of a sensation along the meridian pathways when they have acupuncture treatment.

Although they are now detectable by electronic machines, the student of acupuncture has traditionally spent a considerable portion of his time learning to locate the exact position of the approximately 365 points on the meridians. The points are very small (about 2.5 mm in diameter) and for the full effect of intervention to be realized it is necessary to be extremely precise in their location. Many of the most commonly used points are located on the limbs, below the elbow and the knee, and much of the treatment will take place on these points regardless of the location of the symptom.

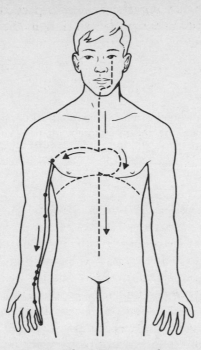

Fig. 2. The Heart Meridian

These pathways of Qi running throughout the body are known as meridians or channels. Each meridian is linked with a particular organ and is responsible for many functions in our bodies, minds and spirits. The meridians can be compared to the major blood vessels in the sense that they constitute the main 'arteries' of energy in the body; but just as tiny capillaries carry blood to every cell in the body, so also there are tiny channels to transport Qi to every cell. Without Qi and blood a cell will die.[6] In modern times hundreds of 'new' points have been discovered on these smaller channels and many of these are used for local symptomatic relief.

When the acupuncturist inserts a fine needle into one of the acupuncture points of the body, he influences the Qi according to the nature of that particular point and the needle technique used. Treating any point will have an effect upon the patient's entire body, mind and spirit, but by choosing certain points and using particular techniques, the practitioner can direct his treatment towards a specific level. There are many situations when it is appropriate to orient the treatment exclusively to the physical level. But there are also times when a person, whether he is presenting physical or psychological symptoms, needs treatment at a deeper level if the cause of the condition is to be affected. The *Nei Jing* makes the point in this way:

> Nowadays vitality and energy are considered the foundation of life; in order to keep them flourishing they must be protected and the life-giving force must rule. When this force does not support life, its foundation will dissolve, and how can a disease be cured when there is no spiritual energy in the body?

WHAT DO ACUPUNCTURISTS MEAN BY BODY/MIND/SPIRIT?

The expression Body/Mind/Spirit has become the phrase most commonly used in the Natural Medicines to describe the different levels of the human being. I use it here because of its familiarity and because it expresses reasonably accurately the Oriental view, although it never appears in exactly this form in any of the Classics of Chinese medicine.

What do we mean by Spirit?

This is a difficult topic, largely because many people already have a firm view of what the word means to them and also because this one word has so many different meanings in the English language. The Oxford English Dictionary lists 34 separate meanings but the one that is closest to its meaning in Chinese medicine is 'the animating or vital principle in man'. Cicero called it 'the true self, not that physical figure which can be pointed out by your finger'. When the novelist Thackeray described one of his characters as 'saddened and humbled in spirit' he was describing the very deepest essence in a person. In the *Nei Jing*, Qi Bo the acupuncture master says:

> What is the spirit? The spirit cannot be heard with the ear. The eye must be brilliant of perception and the heart must be open and attentive, and then the spirit is suddenly revealed through one's own consciousness. It cannot be expressed

through the mouth; only the heart can express all that can be looked on. If one pays close attention one may suddenly know it but one can just as suddenly lose this knowledge. But the spirit becomes clear to man as though the wind has blown away the cloud.

The acupuncturist's ability to perceive the nature of the imbalances in a person's spirit is the acme of the art of acupuncture.

Often people equate 'spirit' with the spiritual and religious sides of the person. The word 'spirit', however, encompasses many other aspects of being. Religion, mysticism and spiritual awareness emanate from the human spirit but, in the framework of Chinese medicine, so also does the desire to look at a radiant sunset or to listen to uplifting music. When we wake up and experience the joy of seeing a beautiful day dawning, it is our spirit that is touched by that experience.

The Chinese considered that the emotions emanate from a person's spirit. One of the great advantages of this system of medicine is that it enables the practitioner to help a fearful person, a grief-stricken person, a resentful person or a person who rarely feels joyful. Acupuncture strives to free the individual from being dominated by a particular emotion or being impoverished by the lack of an appropriate emotion.

Emotions also constitute the 'internal causes of disease' as, when they become extreme, they create imbalances in the healthy functioning of the person's Qi. If the Qi of one's spirit is no longer healthy and vital then the imbalance may spread and manifest symptoms on any level of body, mind or spirit. This is probably the commonest cause of chronic illness. The *Nei Jing* states, 'In order to make acupuncture thorough and effective, one must first cure the spirit'.

The English language has a variety of words to describe the states which arise when one's spirit becomes distressed: despairing, apathetic, paranoid, cut-off, insecure, desperate, depressed, anxious, vulnerable, resigned, bitter, self-centred, lacking self-esteem, etc. These are powerful words but they describe how many people feel for much of their lives. Cicero observed that 'Diseases of the soul are more dangerous and more numerous than those of the body'.

The Chinese regard the health of the person's spirit as

crucial to his health and his chances of recovery. One can often see two people with similar symptoms but they are reacting very differently. One may be at the end of his tether while the other remains inwardly calm. As the *Nei Jing* says 'When the spirit is peaceful, suffering is minute'.

What do we mean by Mind?

What is meant is the cognitive faculty and the ability to think. The phrase 'mentally ill' is legitimately used in Western medicine to describe problems in sense perception, personality, emotions or behaviour. This is a far wider definition than is meant by the word 'mental' in the Chinese medical context. Many people in psychiatric hospitals have extremely astute and able minds, in the language of Chinese medicine it is their spirits that are in distress.

In the context of acupuncture, symptoms on the mental level include a person being obsessed, forgetful, indecisive, unable to concentrate, disorganized, muddled, vague, inarticulate, dyslexic etc.

Although the Chinese acknowledge the importance of the brain in the functioning of the mind, they also consider the mind to be an aspect of the person's Qi. Just as Qi is present in every cell in the body, so also is the person's mind and spirit.

What do we mean by Body?

This, of course, is the least ambiguous of the three levels. When most people in the West think about their health, they think almost exclusively about their physical health. Acupuncture has become well-known in the West for its effectiveness in treating a wide range of physical complaints, perhaps above all for its efficacy in reducing or eliminating pain.[7] It is striking, however, that when patients discover that acupuncture can bring about an improvement in how they feel in themselves, how often they regard their overall sense of well-being as their main priority. There is an increasing recognition that physical symptoms are integrally related to the state of health of one's mind and spirit. This is one of the great lessons that the West can learn from the East. Any comprehensive system of medicine must strive to be a therapy that treats at the heart of the individual's illness. Unless it has a clear vision of how the body, mind and spirit interact with each other, then it is doomed to be forever limited to a therapy of symptomatic relief.

2

The Philosophical Basis
Of Chinese Medicine
The Dao, Yin/Yang And
The Five Elements

THE DAO

THE NEI JING, the most important treatise on acupuncture, was written sometime around 200 BC. In the form of a dialogue, it harks back to 'ancient times' when, according to the Yellow Emperor, people enjoyed better health and greater longevity. The Yellow Emperor asks the acupuncture Master, Qi Bo, 'Is this because the world changes from generation to generation? Or is it that mankind is becoming negligent of the laws of nature?' Qi Bo answered 'In ancient times those people who understood the Dao [previously spelt Tao] patterned themselves on Yin and Yang.'

Long before the *Nei Jing*, the Chinese had evolved the philosophy of the Dao (Dao is untranslatable but it is best rendered as the 'Way' or 'Way of Life'). To live in harmony with the Dao was regarded as essential if the human being was to realize her full potential during her time on Earth. Qi Bo continued

There was temperance in eating and drinking. Their hours of rising and retiring were regular and not disorderly and wild. By these means the ancients kept their bodies united with their souls, so as to fulfil their allotted span completely, measuring unto a hundred years before they passed away. Nowadays people are not like this; they use wine as beverage and they adopt recklessness as usual behaviour. They enter the chamber of love in an intoxicated condition; their passions exhaust their vital forces . . . they do not know how to find contentment within themselves; they are not skilled in the control of their spirits . . . For these reasons they reach only one half of the hundred years and then they degenerate.

If this was so in 200 BC it is probably best not to think what Qi Bo would make of our life-styles in the late twentieth century!

We each have to discover our own path to finding 'contentment in ourselves'. Neither Chinese medicine nor Chinese philosophy offers any universal answer to this central mystery of the human condition. They both stress, however, the importance of living in harmony with the Dao and the necessity of living in accordance with nature and the passing of the seasons. No system of medicine in the world can ever fully compensate for the distress in body, mind and spirit that is the inevitable result when a person's life strays too far from the Dao. The role of the acupuncturist is to help to restore the patients' health and enable them to live a little closer to the Dao.

How can we, with our twentieth-century life-styles, live more in tune with the Dao in order to maintain better health? The Chinese believe that we should balance activity with rest, excitement with reflection, that we should conserve our energy in the autumn and winter to balance increased activity in spring and summer. Acupuncturists see many patients whose health has suffered because of their failure to balance these aspects of their lives. One sees workaholics who scarcely rest, whether they are ambitious businessmen or housewives. Children become ill because they study hard for their exams and then 'relax' in front of the television, thereby failing to balance the mental strain with the physical activity which is so essential for children. Many people suffer ill-health when they retire from their jobs and then do not find satisfying activities to replace their former employment.

In order to further their understanding of the Dao, the Chinese developed two concepts which together form the basis of Chinese medical theory; Yin/Yang and the Five Elements. Both these ideas pervade Chinese thought, not just in medicine, but also in politics, science, art and religion.

They are metaphors to describe how phenomena in nature function in relation to each other. The Chinese observed that in nature there is constant change and their finest physicians created a system of medicine that explained how these patterns of change could become imbalanced and produce illness in a human being. The truths expressed in these concepts are universal; they apply equally to patients in the East and West and are as valid today as they were 3000 years ago.

YIN/YANG

The *Nei Jing* says 'If Yin and Yang are not in harmony, it is as though there were no autumn opposite the spring, no winter opposite the summer. When Yin and Yang part from each other, the strength of life wilts and the breath of life is extinguished.' In Yin/Yang theory all phenomena are viewed as consisting of varying degrees of Yin and Yang. Yin and Yang are not substances, but are an expression of the two poles of a fundamental duality that exists in nature.

The Chinese ideograms for Yin and Yang depict the dark and sunny sides of a hill. Yin and Yang are constantly in transition, just as in nature day and night constantly change into one another. Night is predominantly Yin, day predominantly Yang.

If you think about a 24-hour cycle you can get some sense of how the Yin/Yang balance changes as the day progresses. At dawn Yin/Yang are in equilibrium. Yang then starts to increasingly predominate until the period of maximum Yang at the height of the day. Yang then declines until equilibrium is again reached at dusk and continues to decline until the period of maximum Yin is reached in the depths of the night. This dynamic is also affected by the balance of day and night according to the changing Yin/Yang nature of the seasons. Winter is predominantly Yin, summer predominantly Yang. However even on mid-summer's day there is a short period of darkness; an interval of Yin within the Yang.

By extension, rest corresponds to Yin, activity corresponds to Yang. Mid-winter is the period of greatest rest in nature, mid-summer the period of maximum activity. Yang also constantly changes into Yin, summer turns to winter, day becomes night, activity must be followed by rest. The famous Tai Ji symbol illustrates how Yin and Yang comprise the whole of creation, how they flow into one another and how there is always Yin within Yang, Yang within Yin.

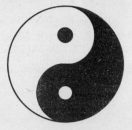

Fig. 3. Yin and Yang Symbol

The following is a list of correspondences of phenomena in nature according to their Yin/Yang nature:

YANG	YIN
Light	Darkness
Activity	Rest
Heaven	Earth
Energy	Matter
Expansion	Contraction
Rising	Descending
Male	Female
Fire	Water

In the Classic known as the *Liu Tzu* it says

> When the Yang has reached its highest point the Yin begins to rise, and when the Yin has reached its greatest altitude it begins to decline, and when the moon has waxed to its full it begins to wane. This is the changeless Dao of Heaven. After the year's fullness follows decay, and the keenest joy is followed by sadness. This is the changeless condition of Man.

How does the theory of Yin/Yang apply to Acupuncture?

According to the *Nei Jing* one of the principal tasks of the acupuncturist is to 'observe the relationship between Yin and Yang carefully, and to make adjustments to bring about equilibrium'. In order to do this she must assess various factors in her diagnosis of a person's Qi, according to their Yin/Yang nature. The following are a few examples:

YANG	YIN
Fire	Water
Heat	Cold
Dry	Wet
Hyper-active	Hypo-active

Fire/Water

The juxtaposition of Fire and Water may seem strange unless one bears in mind that Fire represents the flame that keeps alive and stokes all metabolic processes. Our bodies need to be kept constantly within a degree or two of 36–37 Celsius in order to function at their best.

Water constitutes over seventy-five percent of the human body and is essential to moisten and cool the body's physiological functions, to balance the warming action of the Fire. If this balance becomes disturbed then the body's functioning is inevitably affected. If the fire becomes weak then the water will start to be in excess and the body's metabolism will become unable to carry out the many functions necessary to ensure health. If the water becomes deficient then the fire will start to rage out of control. The phrase 'Gung-Ho' entered the English language from Chinese medicine where it is used to describe somebody when the Fire of her Liver (Gan = Liver; Ho = Fire) is in excess, leading to a red face, quick temper and generally a 'Gung-Ho' attitude to life!

Heat/Cold

An acupuncturist can learn a great deal about the Yin/Yang nature of a person from whether she feels the cold excessively, finds hot weather difficult to deal with or copes well with either extreme. Acupuncturists see many patients who are always trying to keep themselves warm, snuggling up to fires, cuddling hot-water bottles and dreaming of holidays in the sun. These people are basically deficient in Yang and part of their treatment will concentrate on strengthening and warming the more Yang aspects of their Qi. Moxibustion, which involves smouldering small quantities of a herb on acupuncture points, is often used for this purpose.

It is also possible to apply the criterion of heat/cold to specific symptoms; for example many painful joints, often given names such as arthritis, rheumatism or lumbago in the West, are cold to the touch and feel less painful after a hot bath or when other forms of heat are applied. Many, however, are unaffected or made even more painful by heat. For the acupuncturist it is obvious that this is a different syndrome and will require different treatment.

When too much heat is present in the body there will be a tendency for the person to have scanty and dark urination, constipation, a red complexion, a red tongue and in acute cases, fever. Conversely if there is too much cold the person will be prone to profuse pale urination, loose stools, a pale face and a pale tongue.

Dry/Wet

Dry eyes, dry skin, dry stools, a dry cough and any other symptoms of dryness all indicate an excess of Yang in the body. Swollen ankles, excessive sweating, frequent urination, a runny nose or any other symptoms of excess wetness indicate an excess of Yin in the body.

Hyperactive/Hypoactive

If the person has a tendency towards restlessness, insomnia, rapid speech and movements or emotional volatility then their Yang is probably overwhelming their Yin. If they tend towards lethargy, sleepiness, slow speech and movements or an unemotional phlegmatic temperament then their Yin is predominantly in excess. For example a rapid heart beat probably indicates excess Yang of the Heart, whereas a slow heart beat may indicate excess Yin of the Heart.

The Four Varieties of Yin/Yang Imbalance

Yin and Yang are in a constant state of change but in good health a balance is always maintained. Ill-health will only result when one side starts to 'consume' the other. The

Nei Jing states 'Yin in excess makes Yang suffer; Yang in excess makes Yin suffer. A preponderance of Yang leads to heat manifestations; a preponderance of Yin brings on cold.'

Figure 4 shows in a very simplified form the four basic types of Yin/Yang imbalance.

These four varieties of imbalance require radically different

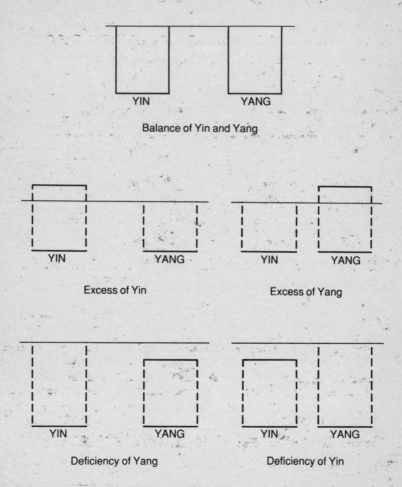

Fig. 4. The four basic types of Yin/Yang imbalance

treatments. These will also be determined by many other factors not least by consideration of the other fundamental axiom of Chinese medicine: the 5 Elements.

THE FIVE ELEMENTS

In the *Nei Jing* the master practitioner Qi Bo expressed the theory in this way:

> The five Elements are Metal, Water, Wood, Fire and Earth. They alternate in succession between a position of pre-eminence and one of insignificance. This transformation provides us with an understanding of life and death, an insight into creation and decay . . . and the times when an illness is minor or serious.

The theory of the 5 Elements is probably not as old as Yin/Yang, although it was certainly in existence by 1000 BC. Each Element is associated with a particular season: Water with winter, Wood with spring, Fire with summer, Earth with late summer and Metal with autumn. Each element represents a different quality in the human being, just as each season brings a different quality to the entire natural world. Spring (Wood) and summer (Fire) are predominantly Yang, autumn (Metal) and winter (Water) predominantly Yin. 'Late summer' (Earth), that is August and September in Britain, is the period when the annual cycle pauses, balanced between the active, growing, Yang phase of the year and the declining, resting, Yin phase.

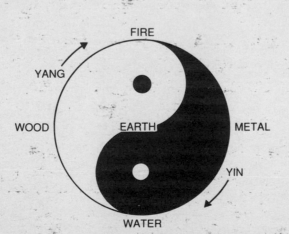

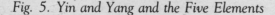

Fig. 5. Yin and Yang and the Five Elements

The 5 Elements (sometimes translated as the 5 Phases) are often depicted as in Figure 6 in order to show the nature of their inter-relationships. Each Element is generated by one and generates another, just as spring requires the resting period of winter in order to come into being and it, by virtue of creating an explosion of growth, enables summer to arrive.

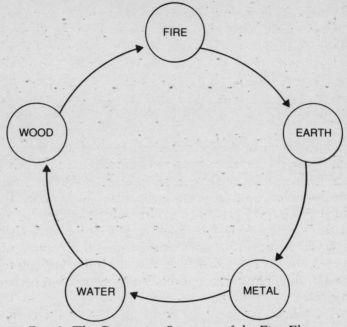

Fig. 6. The Generating Sequence of the Five Elements

How does the theory of the Five Elements apply to Acupuncture?

Essential to the theory of the 5 Elements is the concept that when any of the Elements become distressed, it will lead to some degree of imbalance in the Qi of the body, mind or spirit. Depending on the degree of imbalance within the 5 Elements, this may be mild or may be the cause of severe illness.

Most patients visit an acupuncturist with symptoms stemming from various Elements. The practitioner has to make a diagnosis of the condition of each of the Elements in order to understand the disharmony in the balance between them. This is essential in order to perceive which Element is primarily in distress and which are now struggling due to the initial imbalance. Practitioners who focus much of their diagnosis and treatment on the person's spirit will always try to perceive how the Elements are reflected in the person's character and life.

In diagnosis of the 5 Elements the ability of the practitioner to perceive and assess the emotional nature of the person is crucial, especially in relation to the key emotions of anger, joy, sympathy, grief and fear. Perceiving which emotions have become inappropriate, too intense for the situation or conversely too suppressed, enables the practitioner to discern where the hub of the imbalance in the person's spirit lies.

In the Chinese medical texts there is a great deal of theory to explain how the 5 Elements interact and influence each other. Once there is any degree of imbalance in any Element then some disturbance will occur throughout the entire cycle. The natural process of beginning, growth and flowering, harvest and then storage cannot be fulfilled. Just as the farmer will not see an abundant harvest in the summer if the spring was too cold, too dry or too windy, so also the individual will not have a healthy Fire Element if the Wood Element has become distressed.

What follows is a brief description of some of the characteristics of the 5 Elements with examples of just a few of the ways in which dysfunction of an Element may manifest itself in the temperament of the person.

Wood

Wood is the Element associated with spring; the season of dynamic growth and activity. *It is responsible for initiating change, guiding our development and granting us our ability to mature.* When the Wood Element has become weak the person is often unable to generate the changes necessary to make the circumstances of her life more satisfying and rewarding. Thus, many people's lives become barren and a source of regret and frustration.

The Wood Element also gives us the ability to assert who

we are to the rest of the world. A child draws upon this Element as she grows up and asserts her own uniqueness in relation to her parents. A common way for the Wood Element to become imbalanced is when parents overly repress the assertive sides of their child's character, thereby making it extremely difficult for the child to grow into full adulthood, relatively free from the shadows of her parents' personalities. At the opposite end of the spectrum however, it is just as destructive to a child's Wood for parents to fail to set limits to the assertive demands of a child, thus creating a tyrant instead.

One expects to see a person with a healthy Wood Element develop and 'grow' in herself in harmony with the passing of the years. Just as one can sometimes say that a child is 'young for her age', in the sense that she has not matured alongside her peers, one also sees adults who have not asserted their individuality and achieved maturity in themselves.

Anger is the emotion associated with Wood. Disharmony in the Wood Element itself, and in its relationship to the other Elements, can result in a person becoming inappropriately angry. At the other end of the spectrum, some people with an imbalance in Wood become un-assertive and unwilling to provoke any situation which might produce conflict. How we respond in a situation when anger arises in us is shaped by the health of our Wood Element. This is dependent on the long-term strength of the Element and on the vitality of its Qi at that particular time.

Many people, whether in the realm of career, marriage or family, 'lose their way' at some stage of their lives and find themselves in a situation where their creative and assertive aspects cannot find expression. Their lives stagnate rather than evolve in response to their own changing needs. Frustration, fury, irritability, resentment and despondency are commonly the result.

This is the cause of so much suffering that it often results in the person generating a physical symptom. To treat the symptom alone, without attempting to resolve the underlying emotional cause, may be superficially effective. Often, however, it merely serves to suppress the emotion's physical manifestation. The symptom will probably re-appear at some later stage or, more worryingly, the underlying emotional disharmony will create a more serious illness.

Fire

The predominantly Yang Element of Fire is linked to the season of summer; the time for flowering, warmth and abundance in nature. Whereas the Wood Element is largely concerned with the qualities in ourselves that we need in order to assert our individuality, the Fire Element is mainly responsible for the qualities we draw upon to relate to and bond with other people. Loneliness has always been a feature of many people's lives and it is now reaching epidemic proportions in twentieth-century Western society. However many people they know and however much time they spend socializing, many people still find themselves feeling 'lonely in a crowd', longing for an intimacy that seems to elude them. As the psychiatrist Erich Fromm said 'Many people think that the problem of love is the problem of an *object*, not the problem of a *faculty*. People think that to love is simple, but that to find the right object to love – or to be loved by – is difficult.' For many of our patients their Fire Element has become weakened in such a way that they have become unable to fully give and receive love, often living in loveless marriages or isolated singleness.

The reasons for this usually go back to childhood when many children start to close their hearts in reaction to feeling unloved. Nothing is more devastating to an individual's Fire Element than the experience of being rejected or unwanted. Many children lose strength in their Fire if they *feel* themselves to be unloved, irrespective of how much their parents adore them; for example after a younger sibling enters the family and ousts them from their position of being the sole recipient of their parents' affection.

The Fire Element is responsible for giving us our sparkle, our joy, our warmth. When someone's Fire is low they usually radiate little joy in their voices, their demeanour, their work and their relationships. After receiving treatment on the Fire Element, many patients feel their capacity for joy returning closer to its full potential.

Joy is an emotion predominantly shared with others and some people with imbalances in their Fire Element will often try to stimulate jollity in social situations as a contrast to the rather joyless state that they are often in when they are alone. 'The tears of the clown' may be a cliché, but it symbolizes the emptiness many people feel behind their jolly façade.

Some people with imbalance in the Fire Element, however, are extremely joyful people. The Chinese have always regarded being excessively joyful as being just as imbalanced as being lacking in joy. It may be an 'imbalance' to the acupuncturist but the other side of the coin is that many people with imbalances in Fire have a wonderful ability to be joyful and to bring joy to other people when a situation draws out their sparkle and warmth.

Earth

The Element Earth, balanced in terms of Yin/Yang, is associated with late summer; the season of harvest, when the time of flowering is over but nature has not yet started its phase of decline. It is responsible for giving the individual stability, the ability to adjust to differing circumstances and to cope, whatever the difficulties. A person with a strong and stable Earth Element will manage to remain relatively composed in situations that would make another person feel insecure. *When the Earth Element is in distress the practitioner frequently discerns an internal insecurity that manifests itself as worry, pre-occupation and, in extreme cases, obsessional thoughts or behaviour.*

An imbalance in Earth will often drive the person to look to other people for support, understanding or sympathy. There is, of course, a part of all of us that wants and needs to feel that other people care about what is happening to us. The acupuncturist will try to discern whether this need has become excessive or alternatively whether the person has closed herself off from other people to such an extent that she can no longer truly give or receive sympathy. When the Earth Element is unstable and the person's feelings of sympathy towards others have become excessive, she may find herself being overwhelmed by feelings brought on by watching the news on television or worrying excessively about situations affecting family or friends over which she has no control.

The Earth Element is also inextricably linked with nourishment, in spirit and mind as well as body. We are all born with a store of Qi but it must constantly be replenished by food and water from the Earth as well as air from the Heavens. Many people consult acupuncturists when they have trouble receiving nourishment, whether physically with symptoms like indigestion or poor appetite, or when they have become disturbed about food at deeper levels within themselves. This can manifest as a tendency towards anorexia or perhaps eating excessively to try to satisfy an emotional part of themselves which is not being nourished in any other way.

In childhood the main source of this nourishment and nurturing is one's mother. When, for whatever reason, a person does not receive enough of this quality of nurturing in her life it is hard for her to have a really healthy Earth Element as an adult. Difficulties in one's relationship with one's mother are a common cause of dysfunction in this Element, whether from not receiving enough mothering or in some cases from receiving too much, i.e., 'smothering'. The practitioner, however, will always bear in mind the whole picture of the person and not leap to facile diagnoses based on one aspect of a patient's life.

The home is also an extremely important source of stability for most people. In some people the Earth Element is imbalanced in such a way as to make them excessively dependent upon their home for a feeling of security, in extreme instances being reluctant to go outside the front door. Minor symptoms often occur when people travel and leave the security of their home behind them. So many people experience disruption in their sleep, menstruation, digestion or bowels when they travel that the often heard justification of 'a change in the drinking water' is not a sufficient explanation.

In summary the task of the acupuncturist is often to strengthen the patient's Earth Element in order to liberate the person from needing to look excessively to outside sources for her own internal nourishment and security. That could be home, family, career status or the oral comforts of food or cigarettes.

Metal

Whereas Earth is associated with receiving Qi in the form of nourishment from food, Metal is the Element responsible for receiving Qi from the Heavens. This source of vitality is crucial, not just physically but also to our minds and spirits. In common with many other cultures the Chinese associate Heavenly energies with a male or Yang figure (God the father), whereas the Earth is perceived as a female or Yin force (Mother Earth).

When someone's relationship with their father, or in some cases father figures, has been problematic the Metal Element often becomes afflicted. Few patients, when asked, say that as a child they felt as close to their fathers as to their mothers. Although most children spend less time with their father than their mother, there is no reason why the quality of time spent together should not enable a satisfying bond to be formed and developed. Many people, however, express the feeling that their father was more distant, more remote than their mother and often feel a sense of loss that the relationship was not closer or warmer. This will not necessarily lead to dysfunction in the Metal Element but when this feeling is strong then it is often indicated.

The Metal Element is linked with the season of autumn; a time of decline when nature withdraws into itself. The emotion associated with Metal is commonly translated from the Chinese as grief, but also such feelings as sadness, melancholy, disappointment and regret stem from the Metal Element. These feelings become excessive or inappropriate when someone's Metal is out of balance with the other Elements and they are commonly experienced during the season of autumn. The overt expression of grief is far more repressed in Britain, where the 'stiff upper lip' is so valued, than in other cultures. For example, it is unusual for people to weep publicly at funerals and it is rare for a person to cry with another person without feeling obliged to offer an apology. One can, however, often detect an intense sense of loss which a person will only express to another person when a very intimate rapport exists. The price paid for denying the expression of this range of emotions is often an inner deadness, a cut-offness or a melancholy depression.

It should be remembered that Metal is predominantly Yin and therefore its expression is bound to be less visible, less on the surface than the more Yang Elements of Wood, Fire and Earth. It is responsible for bringing richness and quality to one's inner life. When this function is weakened the person often finds that her experience of all manner of situations is not satisfying, either in work, socially or in time spent alone. Cynicism, boredom and apathy are the inevitable corollary when life loses its richness. Feelings of inadequacy, guilt, lack of self-worth and an excessively self-critical attitude are common complaints of patients with imbalance in the Metal Element. The acupuncturist in these instances will address much of the treatment to bringing this Element back into harmony with the other Elements.

Water

This is the most Yin Element and often the most difficult to perceive as its role in the spirit of the person is often the least overt. In winter the life-force of nature is at its most latent; the Qi in a seed is fully present but waiting for the arrival of spring to move into a more Yang, active stage. *Water is responsible for our Will, our drive, our ability to realize our potential.* It is described as 'the Foundation of all Yin and Yang energies' and it is this quality of being the foundation for the other phases in the cycle of the 5 Elements which characterizes this Element. There are many people who run on 'nervous energy' when they lack the reserves which should be available to them from a strong Water Element. These people often achieve a great deal as the deficiency in the Yin of their Water gives them a restless, hyper-active quality that means that they are strongly driven by their Will. Many workaholics, entrepreneurs and politicians have this imbalance while people who are deficient in the Yang of their Water tend to be lacking in drive, ambition and vitality. When Water is healthy then the person is neither 'driven' nor lacking in ambition.

Water is also the origin of our congenital 'Essence' (Jing) which determines our basic constitution and our ability to develop from a fertilized egg through the stages of being an embryo, baby, child, adolescent and adult. Although it is hard to bring about a complete cure when a person's constitutional health is weak, acupuncture can still be extremely effective.

If the Water Element is imbalanced then fear is the emotion that becomes excessive or inappropriate. There are times when anxiety, suspiciousness, even paranoia may be justified but many people have become chronically fearful, anxious in situations that do not truly warrant it. This is often hard to detect as most people are loath to reveal their fear to other people. Often it can be detected most easily in the eyes or by body movement. Many people try to still their bodies in order to suppress the intensity of their anxiety whereas other people find it hard to keep their eyes and body still when they are nervous. The acupuncturist, however, must gain some understanding of the nature of a patient's fear if she is to make a diagnosis of the health of the Water Element.

The other side of the coin of fear is excitement and courage. Some people love to put themselves in situations where they become adrenalized because it makes them feel more alive, more vital. Fun-fairs, horror movies, driving too fast or even participating in dangerous activities such as parachuting and rock-climbing are all enjoyed by people who, because of the nature of their Water Element, like to stimulate their levels of excitation. Equally these activities are loathed by people whose levels of excitation are quite high enough already!

Diagnosis of the balance of Yin/Yang and the 5 Elements is crucial to the acupuncturist's understanding of the person and together these two theories form the theoretical basis of acupuncture. In order to make the diagnosis more specific the practitioner must also examine the condition of the twelve separate functions in the body, mind and spirit.

3

The Twelve Meridians

T HE CHINESE DISCOVERED that each of the 12 meridians, the pathways of Qi, is linked to a particular organ. Their concept of an organ, however, incorporates much more than simply the physical structure. *In Chinese medicine an organ is not defined by its structure and location; it is defined by its function.* Not by what it is; but by what it does. The Heart, for example, is considered by an acupuncturist to control the entire vascular system. The Lungs are considered to be responsible for the whole process of breathing, from the nose down through the trachea to the organ of the lungs themselves. Even if an organ is removed, such as the gall-bladder or spleen, the functioning of the meridian still continues.[8]

Apart from its physical functions, each organ is endowed with attributes of the mind and spirit. The *Nei Jing* compares each organ to an official in a Court with each one fulfilling specific functions: one 'is like the minister of the monarch' another 'has the functions of a military leader'. 'These 12 officials should not fail to assist each other' for once one of the 'officials' begins to perform his duties less than adequately, then the other 'officials' will inevitably be affected and symptoms will occur in body, mind or spirit.

Acupuncture works by enhancing the Qi of a meridian so that it can carry out its functions to its maximum potential and thereby resolve whatever symptoms have arisen. Each meridian can only be treated where it runs close to the surface of the skin and this is the pathway that is shown by the solid line on the accompanying diagrams. It also has a deep pathway

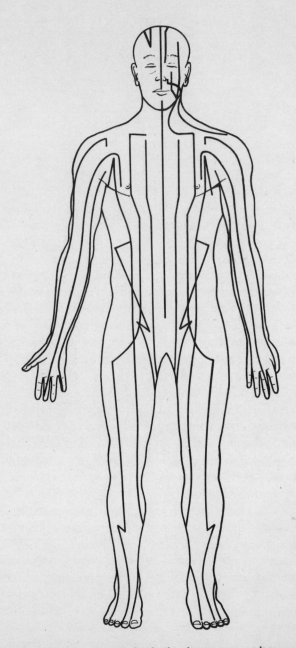

Fig. 7. Front view of the body showing meridian pathways

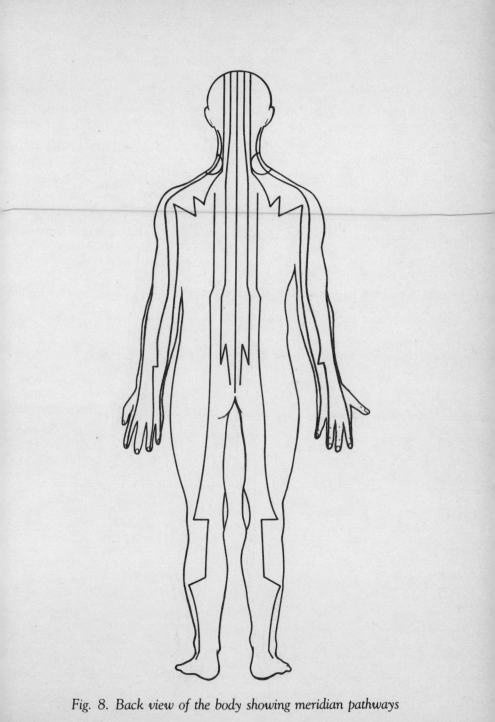

Fig. 8. Back view of the body showing meridian pathways

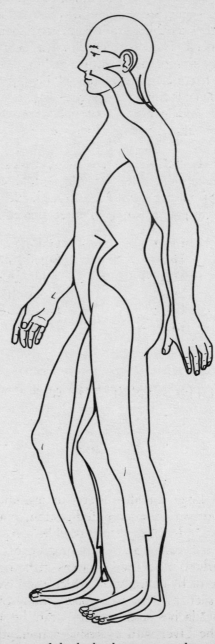

Fig. 9. Side view of the body showing meridian pathways

that travels into the torso and passes through its associated organ. Each meridian has acupuncture points along its pathway, the longest having 67 points, the shortest just 9. Each point has a name: some names describe the point's location, some allude to a quality that treatment of that point can bring to that Official. There is much complex theory to describe the specific functions of each meridian and its associated organ but I am going to concentrate on some of the ways that dysfunction of each Official is commonly seen. *A diagnosis cannot be reached by the simple consideration of symptomatic indications of the officials alone: other diagnostic criteria must always be considered (see Chapter 5).*

Each of the 5 Elements has two Officials attributed to it with the exception of the Fire Element which is responsible for four Officials. The Officials in each Element are closely linked and in practice they are often treated together.

WOOD	Liver	Gall-Bladder
FIRE	Heart	Small Intestine
	Heart-Protector	Triple Burner
EARTH	Spleen	Stomach
METAL	Lungs	Large Intestine
WATER	Kidneys	Bladder

THE OFFICIALS OF THE WOOD ELEMENT

Liver

Body

When the Liver meridian starts to malfunction, digestive disorders are very common. Indigestion, nausea, flatulence and other kinds of digestive troubles can be successfully treated by enhancing the functioning of this meridian. This is particularly so when the symptoms are brought on by eating when tense or by eating foods which the Liver finds hard to deal with such as rich, fatty foods. Many other symptoms, such as headaches and arthritis, can be exacerbated by straining the Liver with excessive consumption of alcohol, chocolate, drugs, cheese, and citrus fruits to name a few of the common culprits. For some people with imbalanced Liver Officials 'excessive' can sometimes mean a tiny amount by other people's standards.

The Liver is one of the most important Officials associated with menstruation, and many types of menstrual problems stem from distress in this Official. Irregular and painful periods, fluid retention and pre-menstrual syndrome can all derive from this Official. Anger is the emotion associated with the Wood Element, so irritability prior to a period is common when this Official is involved.

The Liver has particular responsibility for the functioning of the eyes. If the complaint is either blurred vision, 'floaters' in front of the eyes, dry, sore, tired, or red eyes or any other kind of eye problem, then the acupuncturist will suspect the Liver of being the origin of the trouble.

Mind and Spirit

The Liver Official 'holds the office of general in the armed forces. Assessment of circumstances and conception of plans stem from it.' Its role, as befits an official of the Wood Element, is to initiate action. It is responsible for planning and organizing and the practitioner will attempt to assess these mental faculties. This is partly because they may be deleteriously affecting the patient's life and partly in order to shed light on the condition of this meridian in general. Some people are extremely disorganized, whereas others have everything rigidly planned down to the last detail. An excessive tendency either way is regarded as imbalanced and many people report that they become more efficient after acupuncture treatment on this Official. Certainly the intense pressure of life to-day, cramming far more into each day than ever before, places a great strain on the mental aspects of this Official.

In one's spirit this Official is responsible for giving us our sense of direction, purpose and hope for the future. A practitioner who is adept at diagnosing and treating at this level, is able to enhance these aspects of the human spirit through the use of acupuncture.

Point names on this meridian include Gate of Hope, Spiritual Soul Door and Supreme Rushing.

Gall-Bladder

Body

This Official has manifold functions to perform and, like the Liver, its dysfunction commonly results in problems with digestion, menstruation and the eyes. Its pathway runs from the temples, over the head, down the side of the torso and ends on the feet. Headaches, painful shoulders, arthritic hips and aching knees are frequently the result of distress along the path of the Gall-Bladder meridian. Co-ordination is also the province of this Official and it is noticeable that many women with afflicted Gall-Bladders become clumsy and accident-prone around the time of their periods.

Mind and Spirit

'The Gall Bladder is responsible for what is just and exact. Determination and decision stem from it.' Indecision, confusion, muddle and poor judgement are the result of dysfunction in this Official. These states are particularly evident in people who have strained this organ by smoking cannabis over a long period of time. Cannabis has little effect on the physical level but often saps decisiveness, initiative and clarity in the mind and spirit. The Chinese talk of someone having a 'small' Gall-Bladder when he lacks the personal courage to assert himself and make the decisions that are necessary in his life. The philosopher William James recognized this syndrome when he observed 'There is no more miserable human being than one in whom nothing is habitual but indecision'.

Points on this meridian include Bright and Clear, Eye Window and Sun and Moon.

Case history: Catherine was a woman in her 30s complaining of migraines which were linked to her menstrual cycle. She had suffered from these since puberty but they had become worse since the birth of her children. She had several diagnostic indications, including accident-proneness, irritability, alcohol intolerance and being very disorganized, all of which pointed to the principal problem being in her Gall-Bladder and Liver meridians. She also spoke with some feeling of the fact that as a child and teenager her mother made *all* her decisions for her and that if it was at all possible she still preferred to let her husband make all decisions, important or trivial.

THE OFFICIALS OF THE FIRE ELEMENT

Heart

Body

The Heart is spoken of in the Classics as 'the root of life', 'the Grand Master' of the other organs and as the Official who 'holds the office of Lord and Sovereign. The radiance of the spirits stems from it.' Many Japanese acupuncturists regard the functioning of this Official as so subtle and so powerful that they seldom treat it.

One of its main roles in the body is to 'govern' the Blood and the entire functioning of the vascular system. As you might now have come to expect, the Chinese and the Western perceptions of what 'blood' is and does, are somewhat different. To the acupuncturist Blood is a form of Qi, albeit a dense and material (Yin) one. It is created from the Qi we receive from our intake of food and air and its main functions are to nourish and moisten the body.

It is not uncommon for patients complaining of heart dysfunction, such as palpitations or arrhythmia, to be told by their doctor after an ECG and other tests that their heart is 100% sound. Sometimes this has even been said immediately prior to a major heart attack. How can this be? To the acupuncturist it is obvious that the Heart Qi is in distress in a way that is not discernible to Western diagnosis. Severe heart symptomatology, for example, angina, breathlessness and heart attacks can also be treated on this meridian. The pathway of the meridian runs from the heart down to the little finger and pain along the pathway is often felt when someone suffers from angina.

The Heart also has a particular connection with the tongue and the ability to speak. Various speech defects such as stuttering or even just tripping over one's words can often be treated successfully on this meridian.

As with all the other Officials, it is very common for an acupuncturist to diagnose dysfunction in the Heart Official without the physical organ of the heart being involved. There will be symptoms, to some degree or another, but they may be only in the mind or spirit or in another aspect of the physical functioning of the Heart Official.

Mind and Spirit

This Official is so crucial to the overall functioning of the person's well-being that distress in the mind and spirit of the Heart is particularly devastating. Joy is the emotion associated with this Fire Official and when it is seriously imbalanced, hysteria, manic behaviour and feeling 'out of control' can result as well as severe depression, insomnia and mental confusion.

Points on this meridian include Little Rushing In, Spirit Path and Utmost Source.

Case history: Margaret was a patient who had had a fairly serious car crash several days previously. She was now suffering delayed symptoms from the shock. She was bursting into tears without any provocation, feeling alternately hot and cold, depressed and her mind was so confused that she was barely able to complete a sentence. Acupuncture treatment on one point on the Heart meridian (Spirit Gate) restored her to her normal self by the time she left the clinic.

Heart-Protector

Body

This Official is sometimes known as the Heart-Governor, the Pericardium or Circulation-Sex. Its physical functions are very similar to those of the Heart, in fact many symptoms associated with the heart in Western terms are treated more effectively here than on the Heart meridian itself. The pericardium, the fibrous sheath that surrounds the heart, is governed by this Official and the circulation of the blood is also largely dependent upon its health. As the 'Protector of the Heart' one of its jobs is to bear the brunt of any effects of extreme heat upon the Heart. Treatment on this meridian is often effective after a fever if the person is experiencing difficulty in recovering his former vitality.

Mind and Spirit

This Official is said in the *Nei Jing* to 'guide the subjects in their joys and pleasures'. It controls the person's ability to open and close his 'heart' according to the needs of the situation. Just as this Official protects the Heart physically, it also protects it emotionally and in health gives a person the necessary resilience to suffer the inevitable 'slings and arrows' of life. Some people with damaged Heart-Protectors have closed their hearts to such an extent as to make it virtually impossible for them to enjoy an intimate relationship. In the absence of strong Heart protection they keep people at a distance in order to avoid the possible pain of rejection, the experience of which can be so devastating to one's Heart. But just as there are situations when one needs to have the ability to open one's heart in order to give and receive love and closeness, there are also times when it is appropriate to keep one's heart protected. Some people are inclined to be over-sensitive in non-intimate situations. For example a person, who is inclined to 'wear his heart on his sleeve' often takes it personally if an acquaintance is somewhat abrupt or short, whereas in fact the acquaintance is probably worried about something or just downright hung-over!

'Relationships' are one of the preoccupations of our times and increasingly people are realizing that the problems they experience in forming or maintaining satisfying relationships are due to their own emotional make-up. Good psychotherapy and traditional acupuncture are the most effective therapies I know for bringing about changes in this area.

The physical aspects of sexuality are largely determined by the Kidney Official but the psychological aspects are predominantly affected by the health of the Heart and the Heart-Protector. Sexuality is inextricably linked with intimacy, warmth and love and these qualities are largely determined by the health of this Official. If a person who, because of his excessive vulnerability, becomes withdrawn into himself, then his sexuality will become distorted and a source of discontent rather than a source of happiness and fulfilment.

Points on this meridian include the Palace of Weariness, Heavenly Spring and the Intermediary.

Case history: Robert was a high-powered computer programmer in his late 20s whose main complaint was asthma. He was a good-looking, intelligent and delightful man and potentially a very eligible partner for someone. He had been mildly asthmatic since his teens but it had become significantly worse over the last five years. From his case history it emerged that around that time he had been extremely hurt when his girl-friend had ended their relationship. Since that time he had not had any further sexual relationships and admitted that he did not feel 'strong' enough to enter another relationship. Supported by other diagnostic evidence, treatment was focused on the Heart-Protector. His asthma improved greatly and within a few weeks he initiated a new relationship; a development that he attributed to the changes he felt in himself from his acupuncture treatment.

Small Intestine

Body

Dysfunction of this Official can cause physical symptoms in many different forms. The pathway of the meridian starts on the little finger, runs up the arm, over the shoulder and ends just in front of the ear. Many kinds of musculo-skeletal pain such as frozen shoulder, stiff neck and tennis elbow can be treated successfully on this meridian. Digestive problems, hearing difficulties, tinnitus and urinary symptoms, amongst many others are often caused by imbalance of this Official.

Mind and Spirit

Physically the small intestine is responsible for extracting what the body needs and passing on to the large intestine what is not needed. It is 'responsible for receiving and making things thrive'. In the mind and spirit it performs the same function. This Official is largely responsible for the crucial decisions about what really matters to us, what is pure and what is impure, what our priorities are. When this function is not working well then often the person becomes stuck in ambivalence; unable to commit himself to a career, relationship or any course of action that could be nourishing for him. The person often lacks discernment and discrimination. He tends either to be overly critical and cynical or, at the other extreme, to be naïve and gullible.

Points on this meridian include Nourishing the Old, Listening Palace and Grasping the Wind.

Triple Burner

Body

This Official, sometimes known as the Three Heater, has no physical organ with which it is associated but its functions affect the workings of all the other 11 Officials. It has three separate 'Burners'; the Upper which is located in the chest, the Middle which lies between the diaphragm and the navel and the Lower which is situated in the lower abdomen. These three areas should all be the same temperature to the touch. If one Burner is significantly warmer or cooler than the others then it signifies an imbalance in the functioning of the Triple Burner and possibly therefore of the organs situated in that area of the body.

The Triple Burner is essential to balance the Fire and Water, the Yang and the Yin, in the body. It 'is responsible for the opening up of passages and irrigation' and acts as a thermostat in the body, regulating our body temperature as the temperature outside changes. If Yin is deficient the body

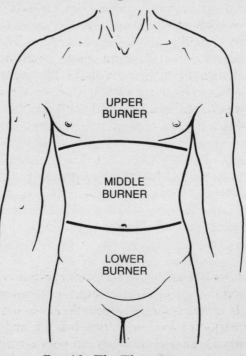

Fig. 10. The Three Burners

will either start to overheat in some area and dry up some of the necessary fluids or conversely if Yang is deficient it will become too cold and inert with a consequent increase in fluids. This Official is therefore of crucial importance in the treatment of fevers and chills and also when someone loses the warmth of his body when he becomes ill or tired.

Mind and Spirit

The Triple Burner is important for its role of regulating the stability of the Fire Element. The person is inclined to be excessively volatile or extraordinarily phlegmatic if this Official is imbalanced. It also plays a part in our relationships with other people but in a far less intimate way than that Heart-Protector. One's ability to deal with non-intimate contact, such as in groups of people, is partly dependent on the Triple Burner. This explains why some people are so adept at being the life and soul of the party yet find one-to-one relationships problematical, whereas other people maintain very loving intimate relationships but are ill at ease in a room full of people.

Points on this meridian include Branch Ditch, Heavenly Well and Assembly of Ancestors.

Case history: Jennifer suffers from multiple sclerosis which has always been far more limiting during either hot or cold weather. Although she still has the illness, treatment primarily on her Triple Burner has improved the quality of her life a great deal and has mitigated the devastating effects of extremes of heat and cold.

THE OFFICIALS OF THE EARTH ELEMENT

Spleen

Body

The Spleen Official encompasses a far wider range of functions than those performed by the spleen organ in terms of Western physiology. It is closely linked to the Stomach and assists in the transformation of food and drink into Qi and Blood. It also distributes Qi around the body, so poor circulation and heavy-feeling limbs are often the result of Spleen dysfunction.

It is noticeable that, in general, women are more prone to cold extremities than men. This is because menstruation is largely dependent upon the Spleen for its healthy functioning and this places more of a strain on this Official in women than in men. Interestingly several points on this meridian are commonly tender to the touch on women.

The Spleen also controls the condition of the flesh and muscles. Many people find that, under the stress of their busy lives, their muscle tone becomes increasingly tight. As a consequence, they experience stiff necks, tense shoulders or an aching lower back. Many 'slipped discs' and dislocations of the spine and neck are caused by the musculature becoming unable to respond effectively to the strains imposed upon it in daily life.

The Spleen has such a wide range of functions to perform that a huge variety of physical symptoms can arise when it becomes imbalanced. Fatigue, obesity, digestive problems, diarrhoea and prolapses are some of the most frequently seen.

Mind and Spirit

Thoughts, ideas and opinions are largely dependent upon the Spleen for their creation and resolution. The tendency when one's Spleen is imbalanced is for one's thoughts to go round and round over the same ground or, as the Chinese rather sweetly put it, to 'think too much'. Worry is the bane of many people's lives, preventing them from sleeping well and unnecessarily occupying much of their waking thoughts. At worst, imbalance of the Spleen can lead to pre-occupation, obsessions and compulsive behaviour. As the Marquess of Halifax, the politician and man-of-letters, said 'A man may dwell so long upon a thought that it may take him prisoner'.

Points upon the Spleen meridian include Earth Motivator, Encircling Glory and Sea of Blood.

Stomach

Body

This Official carries out the first part of the process of receiving food and drink into our bodies and transforming it into Qi. It is responsible for the entire food pathway from the saliva in our mouths, down through the oesophagus and into the stomach and duodenum. Along with the Spleen it is 'responsible for the storehouses and granaries', regarded as one of the most important positions in a country stalked by famine throughout history. 'Have you eaten to-day' is a common greeting in China and this phrase reflects a still evident Chinese concern about food and the state of their digestion.

The Stomach must 'rot and ripen' the food and drink and this, along with the functioning of the Spleen, determines the condition of one's digestive metabolism. People with the largest appetites are often as thin as rakes and conversely some people seem to put on weight just by 'looking at food'. When this rotting and ripening function does not work well, symptoms such as indigestion, belching, obesity, ulcers, bowel problems and a general lack of vitality are frequently the result.

Mind and Spirit

So many people in our society have some difficulties in their attitude towards food. Media and peer pressure to be thin often conflicts with the abundant availability of foods almost guaranteed to make one fat. This makes it very hard for many people to maintain a healthy attitude to food. Comfort-eating, bingeing, poor appetite and a general pre-occupation with food are very common and often respond well to treatment on this Official.

The ability to assimilate new ideas, concentrate and absorb information is also the province of this Official. If while reading a page of a book you realize nothing has gone in, then your Stomach Official is probably not at its best!

Points on this meridian include Abundant Splendour, Heavenly Pivot and People Welcome.

Case history: Anna is a University lecturer in her mid-50s who came for acupuncture treatment primarily for her arthritic knees. The case history also revealed menopausal problems such as hot flushes and excessive mood swings, a stomach ulcer, insomnia, a tendency to eat too much, feelings of tiredness and cold extremities. Her mind was exceptionally creative but she reported that she found it hard to 'switch it off' and generally found it difficult to relax. Treatment, primarily centred on her Spleen and Stomach meridians, brought about an improvement in all her symptoms. She still comes for treatment once or twice a year to prevent any form of relapse and also to prevent the onset of any new symptoms that might arise from her stressful job and family life.

THE OFFICIALS OF THE METAL ELEMENT

Lungs

Body

The Lungs 'govern the breaths' and they are commonly treated when a person suffers from symptoms such as asthma, emphysema, bronchitis or other lung problems. They are also largely responsible for the production of 'Defensive Qi' which protects us from external climatic factors, such as wind and damp, to which the Lungs are especially vulnerable. Treatment on this Official is often effective at reducing a person's susceptibility to infections of the sinuses, throat and chest.

The Lungs also largely govern the condition of the skin. The link between skin and lung problems is well known to Western medicine; for example it is common to see children develop asthma if they use suppressive treatments, such as hydrocortisone cream, for their eczema. The Lungs play a crucial role in the regulation of fluids in the body and when they malfunction, dry or wet skin, oedema, abnormality of perspiration or excessive phlegm are frequently the result.

Mind and Spirit

The Lungs are like 'a Minister from whom policies are issued' and they work directly under the control of the Heart, the Emperor. Their role is to receive the 'Heavenly Qi' and to provide inspiration and a sense of meaning to one's life.

When this Official becomes imbalanced there is a common tendency for a person to become cut-off from new ideas, people and the experiences of life in general. Boredom, apathy, and a feeling that life is passing one by are the inevitable consequence of being unable to let in and 'receive' the richness of human experience. This is sometimes accompanied by a desperate need to enjoy some form of quality, some sense of meaning in one's existence. This may manifest as a search for 'someone who has all the answers', such as a father-figure, a role-model or a guru who will supposedly reveal to the person a depth of wisdom and experience previously unavailable to him. For other people it shows in more mundane ways; being 'successful', driving an expensive car, eating in high-class restaurants, or marrying a partner who will supposedly enhance one's prestige are just a few of the ways that people attempt to compensate for the inner feeling that their lives lack a sense of fulfilment and purpose. As it says in the great Classic of Chinese thought, the *Huainanzi*, 'Instead of bringing joy from inside to outside we have tried to bring rejoicing from outside to inside. The music rings out and we are full of joy but when the tune ends we are distressed.'

Points on this meridian include Very Great Abyss, Heavenly Palace and Cloud Gate.

Large Intestine

Body

The Large Intestine is responsible for the elimination of waste from the body. It may not be a glamorous job but it is essential to the healthy functioning of the body. Waste matter is primarily excreted through the bowel and symptoms such as constipation, diarrhoea, lower abdominal pain and flatulence are obviously common when this Official becomes imbalanced.

The Large Intestine also discharges waste material through the skin. Spots, blocked pores and greasy skin can all result when it malfunctions. Problems of the throat and nose such as catarrh, sinus trouble and an impaired sense of smell may also arise.

Mind and Spirit

The Large Intestine is closely linked to the Lungs and when one starts to malfunction then inevitably it affects the other. When dysfunction of the Large Intestine predominates, the tendency is for the person to be 'cut-off', not because he can't receive but because he can't 'let go'. Resentment, regret, guilt, an inability to forgive and bitterness frequently result and can poison the ability to 'generate evolution and change', which is the role of the Large Intestine.

Once this function becomes impaired then much of the person's experience becomes tainted. It becomes so much easier to see people's weaknesses rather than their strengths, and that the glass is half-empty rather than half-full. Cynicism is the almost inevitable corollary and often the person finds himself in that sad state of being, as Oscar Wilde put it, 'a man who knows the price of everything and the value of nothing'.

Points on this meridian include Warm Current, Welcome Fragrance and Heavenly Vessel.

Case history: Simon is a teacher in his late 20s who came to acupuncture to help him to stop catching so many coughs and colds. Several times a year these would lead to bronchitis. He had suffered from bouts of suicidal depression since his adolescence but felt that his depressions and his chest complaint had been more severe since the death of his dearly loved father when he was 21. Otherwise he was in good health but suffered from acne despite having a good diet. He enjoyed his work and felt that he 'should have everything to live for' but felt stuck in his sadness for reasons that he did not understand. Treatment on both Officials of the Metal Element brought about improvement in all his symptoms and he now comes to acupuncture only if he starts to lose his sense of well-being or occasionally if he happens to develop an acute physical symptom.

THE OFFICIALS OF THE WATER ELEMENT

Kidneys

Body

The Kidneys are the 'foundation of the Yin and Yang' and they give us our foundation by storing the Jing, the congenital essence which we inherit from the sperm of our father and the ovum of our mother. It determines our constitutional make-up, strength and vitality. As Jing is inherited it can never be quantitatively increased but it can be enhanced by acupuncture, herbs and exercises such as Tai Ji Quan and Qi Gong. Jing is responsible for the growth and development of the person, providing the basis for our transition from embryo through birth, childhood, adulthood and old age. If a person inherits a Jing deficiency he will have poor constitutional health and may suffer from specific problems caused by Jing deficiency such as retarded growth, premature ageing or weakness of sexual activity.

I will try to show how the nature of the Yin/Yang balance of the Kidney Official affects the way that the Official exhibits its disharmony. The Kidneys play a major role in the control of fluids in the body, their Yin nature balancing the Yang influence of the Officials of the Fire Element. If they malfunction, the balance between Fire and Water will inevitably be lost and *any* symptom which involves an excess or a deficiency of fluids may result. If the Yin of the Kidneys is deficient then the person will tend to 'dry up' and tend to have symptoms such as dark, scanty urine, constipation, a dry mouth at night and night sweats. If the Yang of the Kidneys is deficient the person will tend to have abundant clear urine, oedema and loose stools.

The condition of the bones and bone marrow is largely dependent on the Kidneys. Brittle and soft bones as well as poor teeth are commonly seen when this Official is in poor condition.

Apart from the symptoms mentioned above, malfunction of the Kidneys can cause a diverse range of symptoms, such as back pain and certain kinds of asthma, and it is frequently the origin of problems with the ears and nervous system.

Mind and Spirit

'The Kidneys are responsible for the creation of power. Skill and ability stem from them.' They provide us with our will power, our ambition, our drive. If the Yang of the Kidneys is deficient then the individual will be inclined to be somewhat overwhelmed by his fear (the emotion associated with the Water Element) and this will erode his motivation and will. His mind may be deep but it will be slow. People deficient in Kidney Yang are inclined to hide their fear behind a superficially calm exterior and this often gives the impression of internal peace, which unfortunately is not the case.

If the Yin of the Kidneys is weak then the person is inclined to be restless, driven by his will and always striving to conquer fresh challenges. His ambition may be excessive but this is the kind of person to have with you in an emergency for he always seems to have reserves to draw upon. His mind is always on the go and his difficulty is knowing how to relax rather than how to motivate himself. Meditation and relaxation exercises are excellent in order to slow the person down if one can get him relaxed enough in the first place!

Points on this meridian include Ambition Room, Spirit Storehouse and Bubbling Spring.

Bladder

Body

The Bladder meridian has the longest pathway in the body, starting in the corner of the eye and then running over the head, passing twice down the back and then running down the back of the leg to the little toe. Symptoms along its pathway are common, including headaches, many kinds of back pain, sciatica and painful knees.

Its main function is to control the distribution of fluids in the body or as the *Nei Jing* says 'it stores the overflow'. Its function is therefore closely linked to the Kidneys and their symptomatology is similar. Cystitis, incontinence, bed-wetting and other problems where there is an excess or lack of fluid are often treated on this meridian.

Mind and Spirit

This Official plays a crucial role in storing our reserves of energy; physical, mental and spiritual. When circumstances such as tiredness or particularly stressful situations force us to draw upon our inner resources, it is this official that holds the necessary reserves. Some people seem to drain their reserves continually, always running on nervous energy, hardly sleeping or deliberately creating stressful situations or melodramas as a way of making the adrenalin pump and making themselves feel more alive.

This Official is also responsible for the flow of thoughts. When you see a person 'drying up' when he attempts to speak

in public, or someone's mind constantly jumping ahead of itself
or yourself then you are probably in the presence of someone
whose Bladder Official is not all it could be!

Points on this meridian include Eyes Bright, Penetrating
the Valley and Uniting Yang.

Case history: Stephen is a local farmer who has branched
out into various activities such as property development and
a thriving farm shop. His main complaint was that he was
excessively irritable, particularly with his family. Superficially
this would point to an imbalance in the Wood Element but it
soon became apparent that anxiety and fearfulness, although
more hidden, were much more predominant. He was beside
himself with fear if the family were even a few minutes
late back in the car and he endlessly created catastrophic
scenarios about his business schemes. He perspired extremely
freely and could hardly lie still on the treatment couch. He
will always be a fearful person, that is his basic temperament,
but acupuncture treatment on his Water Element has made
him far less so and a great deal less irritable.

The 'Curious' Organs

The twelve Officials also control the condition of the 'curious'
organs: the Uterus (the 'precious envelope of life'), Brain,
Bone Marrow, Bones and Blood Vessels.

Dysfunction of any of these organs is treated on the twelve
Officials as well as the two other meridians in the body, the
Conception and Governor Vessels, the reservoirs of Yin and
Yang Qi.

Once any of our Officials or 'curious' organs becomes over-
or under-active then, in time, some degree of ill-health must
result. What causes the Officials to become distressed is the
subject of the next chapter.

4

The Causes Of Disease

WESTERN AND CHINESE medicine have radically different views about how we become ill. In Western medicine, for example, the notion that the emotional life of the person plays a significant role in a person's physical health is still a controversial hypothesis. Because so little is as yet understood about the complex physiological mechanisms operating, physicians in the West have often denied that physical illnesses frequently have a psychological basis. The word 'psychosomatic' has always had pejorative overtones, implying that the patient could get better if only she tried hard enough.

'Stress', however, became a fashionable word in the 1980s to explain the cause of all manner of illnesses and yet the Western doctor's pharmacopoeia did not significantly alter in response to this development. It is a strange paradox that although nowadays GPs often cite stress as the cause of a person's complaint, the main medical text-books do not even list it in their sections on the causes of disease. In Chinese medicine, however, the links between body, mind and spirit have always been recognized and indeed lie at the heart of the system.

Also at the core of the Chinese view of disease causation is the concept of 'invasion' by climatic forces. This is similar to the age-old notion of catching a chill from being exposed to an extreme climate. The common cold, for example, is described as an 'invasion of Wind and Cold'. Attacks on the body by climatic forces are regarded as a common cause of

many illnesses which can often be treated successfully with
acupuncture.

*Fundamental to the notion of invasion by climatic forces is that
they can only get a grip if there is an underlying weakness in
the person's energetic state.* The Chinese have always been
fascinated by the energetic differences between the people
who became ill during epidemics and those who managed to
resist the infection. Much of the emphasis of the physicians
lay in building up patients' Qi in order to resist the infection
or minimize its effects.

One of the fundamental differences between Western and
Chinese medicine is that, in this context, acupuncturists make
little distinction between cause and effect. If the person exhibits the signs and symptoms of 'Invasion by Wind and Cold' it
does not matter if she is convinced that she has not caught
a chill, nor if a Western doctor diagnoses a streptococcal
infection. The diagnosis of 'Invasion of Wind and Cold'
remains the same because it is a description of the symptoms as
well as an explanation of the cause. Even in the case of a cause
of disease unknown to the ancients, such as radiation sickness,
it has been studied and incorporated into the framework of
Chinese medicine. After the atomic explosions at Hiroshima
and Nagasaki acupuncture and moxibustion were found to be
effective treatments for thousands of people.

The Chinese formulated two main categories of disease
causation: external and internal. *The external causes are climatic
and primarily affect the body. The internal are emotional and affect
the mind and spirit in the first instance.*

THE EXTERNAL CAUSES OF DISEASE

Wind

Apparently there are winds that blow out of central Asia
across the plains of China that make the Mistral seem like a
pleasant breeze. Certainly the Chinese are often at pains not
to become exposed to the wind. An early Classic expressed
this preventive measure as 'The sages of ancient times avoided
the evil wind as one would arrows and stones'.

Some people love the wind and find it stimulating and

pleasant. Some have no strong feelings one way or another. Others dislike the wind because it makes them tense or irritable. Wind particularly affects the Wood Element; anger is the emotion that is liable to arise when this Element is strained. In France the Mistral blowing is even given as grounds for clemency in certain court cases. Strong wind makes many people restless or gives them physical symptoms such as headaches or earaches. School teachers are often well aware of how much harder it is to maintain discipline on windy days.

Even draughts and air-conditioning can produce symptoms in someone whose Qi is weak at the time. Wind enters the body through the pores of the skin which is why one should be at pains to avoid draughts or wind after a hot bath when the pores of the skin are open.

Noise is also regarded as a form of Wind. It is noticeable that a person suffering from a headache caused by dysfunction in the Liver and Gall-Bladder Officials is often extremely sensitive to noise. This is a familiar experience for people suffering hangovers from overtaxing the Liver Official the previous night!

Wind is a Yang force that 'injures Yin' and often produces a sudden onset of symptoms, usually in the Lungs in the first instance. The common cold, characterized by a runny, watery nose and lack of a fever is a combination of Wind and Cold. Influenza and other conditions distinguished by fever, perspiration and thick yellow/green sputum are a combination of Wind and Heat. When Wind becomes present more deeply in the body it particularly affects the Liver and Gall-Bladder and often causes tremors, stiffness, itching or pains that move around from place to place in the body.

Heat

Heat is also predominantly Yang and produces symptoms of redness, sweating, fever, scanty urine and thirst. Sunstroke is an obvious example of an 'invasion of Heat' but one can be invaded by Heat in far less dramatic ways. It is noticeable, for instance, that there is often an outbreak of flu when there is an unseasonably warm spell in winter.

When Heat has invaded, the whole body or portions of it

feel or appear hot. The practitioner will pay close attention to any abnormalities in temperature in any area of the body that is producing symptoms.

If Heat affects the mind and spirit it leads in mild cases to emotional distress; in more extreme cases to manic behaviour: for example the delirium that accompanies high fevers or the aggressive behaviour of many 'skid-row' alcoholics (alcohol, especially spirits, tends to create Heat).

Cold

Cold (as one might imagine) is the opposite of Heat. The weather does not have to be exceptionally cold to create an invasion of Cold; a cool breeze on a summer's evening can generate a Cold condition, especially if one is still dressed for the heat of the day. Cold is Yin and leads to an increase of fluids, for example the extraordinary amount of phlegm that one can produce during the acute phase of the common cold. Parts of the body will feel cold, either localized, or over a wider area as is commonly seen with menstrual problems. The use of moxibustion is especially effective in the treatment of Cold conditions.

One's predisposition to succumbing to an invasion of Heat or Cold is largely determined by one's underlying deficiency in either Yin or Yang. People who are chronically Yang deficient are generally prone to Cold conditions and those who are Yin deficient are frequently susceptible to fevers and other Heat symptoms.

Dampness

The concept of Dampness embraces the situation of living or working in damp surroundings as well as the climatic condition of humidity. Few people thrive in a muggy, oppressive climate but some people find it almost intolerable, due to weakness in the Spleen and Stomach. Subtle feelings in many people's bodies give notice of an approaching thunderstorm: a minority will get symptoms such as a headache or an increase in arthritic pain.

Dampness is Yin and tends to produce an excess of fluids especially in the lower half of the body. Oedema of the legs, fluid retention in the abdomen, vaginal discharges and various urinary and bowel symptoms are frequently experienced by people suffering from Dampness. It is usually seen only in people with some weakness in their Spleen Official so it often increases a person's feelings of tiredness and particularly feelings of heaviness in the legs or head.

Dryness

Dryness is the least commonly seen of the external causes of disease, especially in a damp country like Britain. In fact in Britain 'invasion by dryness' is probably as commonly caused by central-heating as by excessively dry weather. Dryness is predominantly Yang and causes symptoms such as dry throat, dry skin, constipation and thirst.

Four Kinds of Pain

Acupuncture is now used all over the world in the treatment of pain, regrettably often by therapists and doctors who have not studied Chinese medicine. A traditional acupuncturist will always make a diagnosis of the underlying weaknesses as well as assessing which of the external causes has invaded the body and 'blocked' the flow of Qi and Blood through the area. This is known as Bi (obstruction) syndrome and includes symptoms such as arthritis, rheumatism, back pain, neuralgia, bursitis and tennis elbow. Bi syndrome can be divided into four categories although two or even three are often seen together. In order to discriminate between them the acupuncturist will also need to consider other diagnostic criteria, such as the pulse and the tongue, which will be discussed in the next chapter.

1. *Wind Bi.* Sore, painful joints which are widespread in the body. The pain often moves from one area to another for no discernible reason. In an acute form it is often accompanied by fever and chills.
2. *Damp Bi.* The joints are achy, stiff, heavy and usually swollen. The pain is fixed in certain joints. People suffering from Damp Bi often experience more discomfort in humid and wet weather. Damp conditions such as

baths, swimming pools or washing up can also exacerbate Damp Bi.
3. *Cold Bi.* The joints are cold to the touch and are greatly improved with heat and aggravated by cold. The pain is severe and fixed and is usually worse with movement.
4. *Heat Bi.* The joints are red, swollen, hot and sensitive to the touch. Hot baths only serve to make the pain worse and there is a tendency for the person's mouth to be dry and her urine to be dark and scanty.

Diet

The Chinese also regard diet as an extremely important cause of illness. Apart from the obvious dietary causes such as eating too much, too little or the wrong things, Chinese medicine also developed a classification of foods according to their effect upon the person's Qi. If one is suffering from a Heat syndrome one should avoid 'hot' substances such as spices, red meats, garlic, ginger, coffee or alcohol. Garlic, ginger, cayenne and cinnamon are all used, however, in Chinese herbal medicine to dispel Cold conditions.

Cold foods such as ice cream, chilled drinks, salads, fruit and yoghurt should be eaten only moderately by people who tend to Cold conditions and definitely avoided during acute Cold illnesses.

Certain foods produce Damp and should be avoided if a Damp condition is present. All dairy products, fried and rich food, fatty meats, peanuts and ice cream will all create phlegm and exacerbate Damp wherever it is situated in the body.

Sex

The Chinese tend to worry about having too much sex, which seems to be the opposite of what many people worry about in this country. It is regarded as a cause of disease for the reason that ejaculation for a man and, to a lesser extent, orgasm for a woman is held to deplete the Kidney Jing. Many men with weak Kidney Qi experience feelings of tiredness after sex and it is definitely men who take the notion of 'excess sex' most seriously in the East. Too many childbirths in too short a time can deplete a woman's Jing in much the same way. The *Classic of the Simple Girl* (Sui dynasty, AD 581–618) gives the following recommendations for the maximum frequency of ejaculation for men.

Age	In good health	Average health
15–20	Twice a day	Once a day
30	Once a day	Every other day
40	Every 3 days	Every 4 days
50	Every 5 days	Every 10 days
60	Every 10 days	Every 20 days
70	Every 30 days	None

This is obviously only a broad guideline and I am sure it should not be taken *too* seriously. Although the *Classic of the Simple Girl* also gives guidelines about what the minimum frequency of ejaculation should be according to age (at 20 every 4 days; at 40 every 16 days; at 60 every 30 days) this issue is seemingly not discussed in modern China. This is consistent with the lack of emphasis in contemporary China placed upon the internal causes of disease, the emotions.

THE INTERNAL CAUSES OF DISEASE

The ancient Chinese regarded the free expression of emotion as fundamental to human existence. As expressed in Ecclesiastes 'To every thing there is a season, and a time to every purpose under the heaven . . . a time to weep and a time to laugh: a time to mourn and a time to dance'.

How do the emotions cause illness in one's body? It can be most clearly seen in the example of an acute situation. If, for example, you become acutely frightened your body immediately produces a huge surge of adrenalin. The effects of increased adrenalin production upon the body have been extensively studied by physiologists. It is well known that there will be an increase in perspiration, heart rate, urination, circulation of blood to the muscles, etc. In short, it prepares the body for physical action. Different people will react differently; one becomes soaked in sweat whereas another is more aware of the increase in her heart rate, but overall the physiological effects are similar. The emotion of fear has pervaded the person's spirit and this has been biochemically manifested in the body. Other emotions also have profound effects upon the body, which you can feel in yourself if you experience any emotion intensely enough.

When the fear-provoking situation has passed, the person's mind and spirit will settle. The body will calm down and physical function will return to a more normal condition. This is the homoeostatic mechanism; the way of nature. For many people, however, fear-provoking situations have been so intense or so frequent that they have been unable to return to their normal physical function. The effects on the body become chronic. In time, illness arises.

Usually small children most closely embody the Chinese notion of emotional health. The easy transition from an emotion such as sorrow or fear to suddenly laughing and shouting is often achieved in a way that is impossible for adults. This emotional freedom is accompanied by a vitality of spirit that makes small children so enriching and enjoyable to be with.

As the child's character becomes more formed by the emotional and behavioural vagaries of her family, the circumstances of her life and her genetic inheritance, so one sees her become unable to move in and out of different emotions so freely: certain emotions start to predominate, others become repressed. The child gradually acquires a predisposition to particular emotions. Even in a small child one can usually perceive that certain emotions are more powerful and intense than others. The child loses inner vitality as her Qi becomes imbalanced. Yin or Yang will start to predominate; one or more of the Five Elements will lose balance with the others. *It is the development of one's temperament which creates long-term constitutional imbalances in a person's Qi.* These imbalances cause one to become, for example, a fearful person, a person chronically lacking joy, unnecessarily irritable or inexplicably morose.

The practitioner must discern the nature of the constitutional imbalances if she is to treat most chronic symptoms at their true origin.

What is very difficult to determine is whether constitutional Qi imbalances are primarily inherited or predominantly acquired in childhood. The 'nature versus nurture' debate will continue wherever people study humanity, whether they are psychologists, educationalists, acupuncturists or anyone interested in the formation of character. The debate is probably irresolvable, but in a sense makes little clinical difference to the acupuncturist. The key task is to diagnose the nature of the person's imbalances and to assist her to achieve a better state of health. The fact that they may be inherited does not mean that they cannot be successfully treated.

In the short term, acute and intense emotional upheaval may bring about a temporary disequilibrium in a person's Qi. Usually one rapidly returns to feeling as one did before the emotions arose but some people never recover their former well-being after a major upset in their life. The death of a spouse is a classic situation when one can sometimes see a person lose the very will to live. One can also see people's health deteriorate as a result of failing to come to terms with stressful situations in their life such as divorce, redundancy, failure in exams or unresolved conflict with somebody close. Each patient has her personal history which has formed her unique personality and created imbalances in the 5 Elements and Yin/Yang.

In the context of the causes of illness, the Chinese narrowed the vast range of human emotions down to seven, but they should not be interpreted too restrictively. Many other emotions could be included under each broad heading; for example irritation, frustration, resentment, fury and bitterness would all come under the heading of anger as a cause of illness. Certain emotions are inclined to affect particular Elements and Officials but it is worth bearing in mind that people by no means always respond to situations as one might expect – for example the emotion of grief is not always the predominant response to the death of a loved one. Profound lack of joy, the need for sympathy and even anger are sometimes felt far more intensely, depending on the long-term imbalances of the person and the nature of her relationship to the deceased.

The list on the following page shows which Elements are primarily affected by each emotion.

Diet, climatic factors, too much (or too little) sex, congenital abnormalities, injury, lack of exercise, exhaustion and various other causes can all be important factors in a person's

Anger	Wood
Joy	Fire
Worry/Pensiveness	Earth
Sadness	Metal
Fear	Water
Fright	Water/Fire

health, but one's well-being in mind and spirit is probably the most important. Henri Amiel, the Swiss philosopher, expressed what most people feel to be true 'Happiness gives us the energy which is the basis of health'.

Anger

Excessive or unresolved anger is particularly injurious to the Liver and the Wood Element. The *Nan Jing*, one of the Classics of Chinese medicine (approximately AD 100), states 'When anger rises to the head and does not descend, the Liver is injured', and in fact headaches are a common symptom brought on by someone becoming angry or, even more commonly, feeling angry but not expressing or resolving it (i.e., the anger 'not descending').

Many of us have difficulties with anger. Some people explode, some feel frightened by the potential of their anger, some can rarely express or even feel their own anger. Aristotle has probably described the problem better than anybody else:

> It is easy to fly into a passion – anybody can do that – but to be angry with the right person to the right extent and at the right time and with the right object and in the right way – that is not easy, and it is not everyone who can do it.

Anger is our attempt to change a situation that we do not like or that we find unbearable. Failure to assert our needs leads to resignation, resentment, frustration or bitterness to some degree or another. The Chinese regard prolonged or unresolved anger as probably the most destructive emotion to our health and this view is echoed by many Westerners who work in the area of psychosomatic health and illness.

Although in this context I have been describing anger as a

cause of disharmony, the emotion can also be brought on as a result of internal disharmony. The effect of alcohol on the liver is notorious for intensifying some people's anger, while some people drink or take other drugs, such as cannabis, to suppress their feelings of frustration and irritability. People who have especial difficulty with anger are particularly advised to avoid excessive consumption of substances which are toxic to the liver such as alcohol, any drugs and, to a lesser extent, chocolate or rich fatty foods.

Joy

It may seem incongruous to list such a pleasant emotion as joy as a cause of disease but both an excess of joy and a dearth are detrimental to the Fire Element and, in particular, the Heart. It has been noticeable in recent years that many of the most famous British comedians – people whose jollity is infectious enough to make millions laugh with them – have died from heart trouble. Many people strive constantly to be jolly as though 'having a good time' were the be-all and end-all of social intercourse and this places a strain on the meridians of the Fire Element. Jean-Paul Richter, the German satirist, was perceptive enough to write 'No-one is more profoundly sad than he who laughs too much'.

Joy is a social emotion. One may be content and happy on one's own, but laughter and joy are usually most evident in the company of other people. Loneliness and isolation can erode a person's joyfulness in such a way as to be deleterious to health. Conversely when a person forms a relationship which brings joy and love into her life, it often reveals the difference that the polarity of unhappiness and happiness can make to a person's health.

Worry/Pensiveness

Worry is frequently the result of dysfunction in the Earth Element and yet it can also be the cause of distress to that Element. Worry can gain a hold in someone's mind; going over the same thoughts over and over again, in such a way as to become damaging to health. Some people almost boast that if they have nothing to worry about they will find something.

One of the commentators on the *I Jing*, the ancient Chinese Classic of wisdom and divination, summed up this syndrome when he wrote 'All thinking that goes beyond the present situation only serves to make the heart sore'.

Over long periods of time or in acute cases, worry can progress to excessive pensiveness, pre-occupation or obsession. Some people become so wrapped up in their thoughts that they find it hard to sleep, to concentrate or to be spontaneous with other people. They become increasingly withdrawn as they retreat into the private world of their own thoughts and concerns. One can see this happen frequently in people whose work requires a great deal of thought or in people who become overwhelmed by their troubles. Worry can lead to depression and anxiety; at worst serious mental illness.

Stomach ulcers (the Stomach is one of the Officials of the Earth Element) are considered in the West to occur commonly amongst people who are prone to worry. Acupuncturists regard ulcers as well as hundreds of other physical symptoms as being often caused by worry. Martin Luther clearly understood the deleterious effects of worry when he wrote 'Heavy thoughts bring on physical maladies; when the soul is oppressed so is the body'.

Sadness

Although Western medicine has no understanding of the physiological mechanisms involved, the fact that intense grief can shatter a person's health is well-known in all cultures. It is entirely natural to grieve over the death of someone one loves, but after a time it is essential to one's well-being that the sense of loss should diminish in intensity. Some people still feel the loss of someone as keenly years afterwards as they did in the first few weeks and months. This may be evident to the outsider, as the person may still be overtly grief-stricken. However, it is probably more deleterious if a person fails to express the emotion. A Turkish proverb says 'She who conceals her grief has no remedy for it' and certainly it is common for physical illness to arise when a person is unable to express or come to terms with her grief.

Sadness sits heavily on many people. A sense of loss, disappointment, regret and melancholia are forms of sadness which can permeate a person's spirit. These are not emotions that are freely displayed to others, but if the practitioner achieves an intimate rapport with the patient it may become apparent that sadness has caused dysfunction in the Metal Element.

Fear/Shock

Fear predominantly affects the Water Element, the Kidney and Bladder Officials. Earlier in the chapter I described how fear affects the body: adrenalin production increases, muscle tone tightens, heart rate and perspiration increase. Bed-wetting amongst children is often an example of a symptom provoked by fearfulness and the escalating spiral of fear leading to tension and pain in childbirth is now receiving much attention.

A sudden fright is very unsettling and can sometimes leave its mark upon a person's Heart or Kidneys, but chronic anxiety is usually far more destructive. Anxiety and fearfulness are extraordinarily unpleasant states as they can permeate nearly all the situations of a person's life, from waking through to sleeping. A Japanese proverb states 'Every little yielding to anxiety is a step away from the natural heart of man', but there often seems to be little an individual can do to overcome these feelings. Fearfulness, like the other emotions, is an aspect of one's spirit and cannot usually be rationalized away by one's mind. For example, in the case of someone who is phobic about spiders it does not matter how often she tells herself that spiders cannot actually harm her, the fear remains just as intense. The feeling of being like a rabbit caught in the headlights, trapped in the dilemma of fight or flight, is played out in subtle ways by millions of people countless times a day.

Fear has a positive side: we all need to exercise caution in the world. Aeschylus wrote 'There are times when fear is good. It must keep its watchful place at the heart's controls.' The more Yang, outgoing, extrovert emotions of anger and joy need to be balanced by the more Yin, personal, introvert emotions of sadness and fear in order for a person to balance the Yin and the Yang inside herself.

Hua Shou, one of the many commentators on the *Nan Jing*, wrote in 1361:

In conclusion, grief, thoughts, rage, anger, drinking and eating, movement and exertion cause harm if they are developed excessively. Of course, man cannot get along without grief, thoughts, rage, anger, food and drink, movement and exertion. If the development of these states remains in a medium range, how could they result in injuries? However in case of excess, harm to man is inevitable. Hence those who are well versed in nourishing their life avoid extremes and exaggerations. They adapt themselves to the mean, and that is sufficient.

The Chinese concept of following the 'Middle Way', avoiding extremes, is fundamental to their view of avoiding illness and promoting longevity. At the heart of their system of medicine lies the realization that imbalance of an individual's emotions inevitably leads to imbalance of physical functioning. Sadly, this truth has almost become lost in the scientific revolution in Western medicine which has taken place over the last century. Yet it has been well known to perceptive observers of the human condition in all cultures, and at all times. Charles Péguy, the French man of letters, maintained 'when a man lies dying, he does not die from the illness alone. He dies from his whole life.'

5

How Does An Acupuncturist
Make A Diagnosis?

OVER THOUSANDS OF YEARS, the Chinese, and subsequently the other nations of the Orient, developed sophisticated forms of diagnosis which gave them great insight into the nature of the patient's energetic disharmony. Some methods of diagnosis are most useful in assessing specific conditions, some for gaining insight into the nature of the person as a whole. It is the diagnostic skills of the practitioner, his ability to discern accurately both the underlying and the temporary imbalances, that largely distinguishes the Master from the tyro.

Before the invention of blood tests, X-rays, ECGs and the other modern diagnostic techniques of Western medicine, practitioners of all forms of traditional medicine had to rely on external manifestations in order to understand the nature of the patient's illness. Hippocrates, writing in Greece at around the same time as the writers of the *Nei Jing*, stated 'In the medical arts there exists no certainty except in the physical senses'. The acupuncturist must work constantly to develop his ability to 'look, hear, touch and smell', for all the diagnostic information he needs is discernible to the senses, if only he has sufficient sensitivity. Much can be revealed to the acupuncturist through his diagnostic methods that remains unseen by the most sophisticated techniques of Western medicine. What is extraordinary about Chinese medicine is that its diagnostic and therapeutic methods are so effective that it continues to enjoy widespread support throughout the East, despite the introduction of modern scientific medicine. This is in almost total contrast to the West where the state of medicine prior to the nineteenth century was such that, with the exception of some herbal remedies, it has been completely superseded.

Although the basic principles of diagnosis laid down in the Classics of Chinese medicine have remained unchanged, many varied styles of acupuncture have developed over the centuries and throughout the many cultures of the Orient and the West. Since the Communist regime came to power in China in 1949, there has been a concerted attempt to standardize the teaching of acupuncture. This standardized system is known as Traditional Chinese Medicine, or TCM, and it is now spreading throughout the world. Other styles, giving emphasis to aspects of Chinese medicine which are not stressed in contemporary China, place different importance upon certain diagnostic and treatment techniques. Practitioners, according to their training, preferences and aptitude, often concentrate on some methods and are relatively unconcerned about others. Few practitioners, for example, are masters of the traditional form of diagnosis by smell, whereas all acupuncturists place emphasis on pulse diagnosis, for it is central to all traditions of Chinese medicine.

No single item of diagnostic information can ever be considered in isolation, for it is fundamental to the nature of Chinese medicine to see the patient as a whole. The acupuncturist must make a synthesis of a mass of diagnostic information in order to decide which Officials are primarily in distress, what is the nature of the disharmony and how it affects the other Officials. In this chapter, I will attempt to give some idea of how an acupuncturist uses the different components of Chinese medical diagnosis in order to assess the balance of Yin/Yang, the 5 Elements and the 12 Officials.

PULSES

Diagnosis of the pulse is regarded as so important that Chinese patients often speak of going to the acupuncturist as 'going to have my pulse felt'. In olden times many women would not allow themselves to be physically examined or even seen by a doctor and instead would proffer their wrist through a curtain so that the physician could make a diagnosis solely using pulse diagnosis.

The *Nei Jing* states 'The feeling of the pulse is the most important medium of diagnosis. Nothing surpasses the examination of the pulse, for with it errors cannot be committed.' This is not literally true, however, as to master Chinese pulse diagnosis is a life-time's work. What the *Nei Jing* means is that if the acupuncturist has the ability to interpret the pulse accurately then he will be able to discern the true state of health of each of the twelve Officials. To do this, considerable experience is required as well as a total concentration of awareness. The Japanese acupuncturist Yanagiya described it thus 'Focus your attention to your finger tips. Do not speak, do not look, do not listen, do not smell and do not think. This is the key principle of pulse diagnosis.'

Chinese pulse diagnosis can hardly be compared to the examination of the pulse in Western medicine which is predominantly concerned only with the speed of the pulse. However, Galen of Pargamum, along with Hippocrates, one of the founding fathers of Western medicine, placed such an emphasis on subtle pulse diagnosis that he wrote eighteen works on the subject and described over one hundred different pulse qualities. The acupuncturist must feel the pulse of the

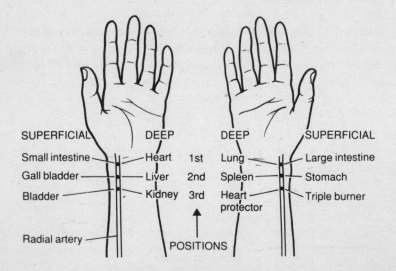

Fig. 11. Pulse Positions

radial artery in six different positions (three on each wrist) and at two different pressures in order to be able to feel the pulse of each of the twelve Officials. To the skilled pulse-taker, this reveals which Officials are relatively healthy and which are imbalanced to such a degree as to be the cause of symptoms for the person.

The Classics describe twenty-eight different qualities which arise in isolation or in combination when an Official malfunctions. These may be present on just one of the twelve pulses or may be on all twelve. To give some examples:

Empty This pulse feels soft and signifies a weakness in the person's Qi.

Full This pulse feels big, strong and hard and denotes an excess of Qi.

Floating This pulse is distinguishable with extremely light pressure. It usually signifies an invasion of an external cause of disease such as Wind, Heat or Cold.

Rapid This pulse has more than 5 beats to the person's breath. It always indicates the presence of Heat. If the pulse is also Empty it means there is a deficiency of Yin; if the pulse is Full it signifies an excess of Yang. This tallies with Western diagnosis where a rapid pulse is used to diagnose a fever.

Slow This pulse has less than 4 beats to the person's breath and (unless the person is an athlete or on certain kinds of medication) denotes a Cold condition. If

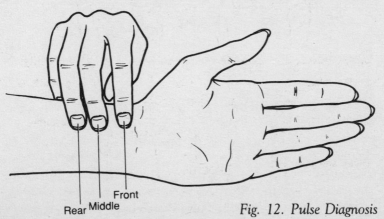

Rear Middle Front

Fig. 12. Pulse Diagnosis

Empty as well it indicates a deficiency of Yang; if Full an excess of Yin.

Slippery Described as like a 'pearl spinning in a dish'. Usually indicates Damp or Phlegm but it can signify pregnancy.

Other qualities include Wiry, Intermittent, Deep, Tight, Hollow, Knotted and sixteen others. As they are often present in combination you may have some idea why pulse diagnosis is regarded as such an extraordinarily difficult skill to master.

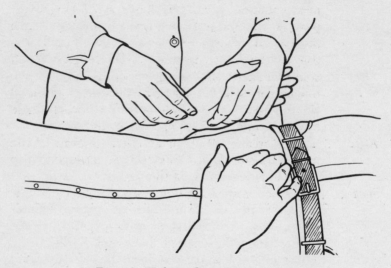

Fig. 13. Taking the patient's pulses

TONGUE

Pulse and tongue diagnosis constitute the 'two pillars' of Oriental diagnosis. In China many teaching establishments have astonishing collections of photographic slides of people's tongues; the more bizarre of which almost defy belief. A great deal of reliable diagnostic information can be gleaned from the tongue as it affords an opportunity to see a part of the inside of the body which otherwise is hidden from the acupuncturist's gaze. Many younger patients in the West are somewhat embarrassed about showing their tongue whereas older patients well remember the time when the doctors would examine their tongue as a routine part of their diagnostic procedure. This has largely fallen out of fashion in Western medicine in line with the decline in emphasis upon examining the appearance of the patient.

In good health the tongue should be pink, moist and with little or no coating. The acupuncturist will examine the tongue for various abnormalities, a few examples of which are listed below:

Colour — Several colours other than pink are possible but most commonly one sees either a red tongue (or parts of the tongue) which signifies the presence of heat (deficiency of Yin or excess Yang) or a pale tongue which usually signifies the presence of cold (deficiency of Yang or excess of Yin). A pale tongue can also be caused by deficiency of Blood which tallies with the Western inclusion of a pale tongue as one of the signs of anaemia.

Area — Various areas of the tongue reflect the state of the internal organs. Figure 14 shows the correspondence of the organs to areas of the tongue:

Shape — A swollen tongue (often characterized by tooth-marks on the sides) indicates an excess of fluids in the body and therefore a Yang deficiency. A thin tongue indicates that the body fluids are being 'burnt up' by the excess heat caused by a Yin deficiency. Other shapes are sometimes seen but less frequently.

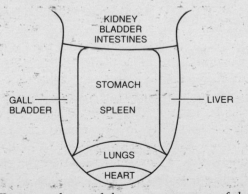

Fig. 14. Correspondence of the organs to areas of the tongue

Coating   The Chinese word for tongue coating can best be translated as 'moss' or 'fur'. It was predominantly the coating on the tongue that the Western doctor used to examine, particularly in the treatment of infection. A tongue coating shows an excess condition: a white coating indicates an excess of Cold – a yellow coating indicates an excess of Heat. This can frequently be seen when there is fever present – try looking at your tongue next time you have the misfortune to have a fever. Cigarette smoking also commonly produces a yellow tongue coating so if a yellow coating is present the acupuncturist will need to enquire whether the patient smokes. Some sweets, soft drinks and fruits can all stain the tongue so the acupuncturist has to keep on his toes! The other common tongue coat is one that is sticky or greasy and this indicates the presence of Dampness or Phlegm.

SPIRIT

The practitioner's assessment of the person's spirit is crucial to his whole understanding of the nature of the person's illness. As the *Nei Jing* says 'If there is spirit the person thrives, if there is no spirit the person dies'. *If the spirit does not 'thrive', then treatment must revitalize the spirit in order to bring about a lasting and profound change in chronic symptoms, whether they are present in the body, mind or spirit.* To determine the vitality of the person's spirit the practitioner must gain a rapport with the patient that transcends the normal social interchange of practitioner/patient relationships. Only when one has, however briefly, contacted the essence which lies behind the 'mask' that a person displays to the world, can one truly make an assessment of whether the spirit 'thrives'.

EMOTION

Although emotions are constantly changing, diagnosis of which emotions are inappropriate, excessive or conspicuous by their absence is crucial to the practitioner's understanding of the patient's constitutional imbalances. One must obviously use great sensitivity to perceive the emotional temperament of the person clearly, as his true nature may well be very different from the characteristics he is prepared to let other people see. De Tocqueville, the great French historian, wrote about one of the emotions:

> I have always thought it rather interesting to follow the involuntary movements of fear in clever people. Fools coarsely display their cowardice in all its nakedness, but the others are able to cover it with a veil so delicate, so daintily woven with small plausible lies, that there is some pleasure to be found in contemplating this ingenious work of the human intelligence.

In the short term also, people have phases of becoming irritable, anxious, lacking in joyfulness, melancholy or being more worried than usual and these may coincide with a deterioration in their physical health or their sense of well-being. Assessing which emotion has become temporarily imbalanced can be a vital diagnostic clue in determining which Official is in distress.

COLOUR

Certain colours in the face will change whenever there is an imbalance of Qi. These are hues that can be seen predominantly on the temples or around the mouth. Each person has a hue; in some people it is quite marked, but in most cases only practitioners who have specialized in this form of diagnosis can discern the colour or combination of colours that indicate the underlying imbalances. In acute cases, however, even lay-people can sometimes see the colours that signify energetic dysfunction. The ashen colour which is common in the event of a heart attack is the same as the 'lack of red' that indicates an imbalance in the Fire Element. The yellow colour that is often noted when somebody feels nauseous is the associated colour of the Earth Element and the Stomach Official. These are just two examples of situations where the early Chinese physicians used their powers of observation to gain insight into the internal functioning of the body. Based upon these perceptions, they formulated their system of medicine.

SOUND

It was also observed that people develop particular tones of voice which reflect underlying energetic imbalances. These may or may not be present in the person's normal voice but will usually become marked when the person becomes somewhat 'charged' with emotion. It is, for example, quite normal for a person's voice to have a slight quality of weeping when he is talking about a situation which has induced sadness. But if you listen closely you can hear that people sometimes have tones in their voices which are not congruent with the emotion they are expressing. They may, for example, have a quality of shouting in their voice when they are being sympathetic or they may laugh when they are describing a situation which has brought them great pain. The inappropriate tone in the voice can give an indication of which Element is primarily in distress.

ODOUR

Many people know and can recognize their own distinctive odour or that of close family members. Many elderly or severely chronically ill people have strong odours. Each person's odour can be classified according to its correspondence with one or more of the 5 Elements. This, like the colour, often changes or becomes more marked when the person becomes acutely ill. The scorched smell of a person with a high fever can be overpowering and TB is an example of an illness that is renowned for giving the person a distinctive odour.

TASTE

Although less reliable than some of the other diagnostic indications, the taste preferences and dislikes of the person may yield information about the balance of the 5 Elements. For example, dysfunction of the Earth Element often predisposes a person to like or dislike the sweet taste. The sweet cravings experienced by many women before menstruation are due to a temporary disequilibrium in their Earth Element. I know a person who used to eat vinegar-soaked bread before she went down with a migraine; the craving for the sour taste being a consequence of the imbalance in her Wood Element. After a course of acupuncture treatment it is common for a person's strong likes or dislikes for certain tastes to lessen considerably.

SEASON

An affinity with, or dislike for, a particular season can also be an indication of imbalance. Some symptoms may only be present at certain times of the year and many people experience profound changes in their sense of well-being during the different seasons. *This is a consequence of the changes in the energetic nature of the macrocosm of Nature, both in terms of Yin/Yang and the 5 Elements. This is inevitably reflected in the microcosm of the human being.* In reasonable health, the person will experience only subtle changes in himself and will be able to enjoy and appreciate each season in turn. In poor health, symptoms such as excessive melancholy in the autumn, chest complaints in the winter or lethargy in the summer may arise.

CLIMATE

Improvement or deterioration in symptoms according to the climate may also provide a clue as to the nature of the imbalance. As outlined in the previous chapter, the climatic forces can be both causes of illness and beneficial influences upon a person's health. For example, to consider two different people with imbalances in their Fire Element; one, with a deficiency in Yin Qi, will probably feel less well in hot weather whereas the other, deficient in Yang Qi, will dislike the cold and look forward to the coming of warmer weather in order to see an improvement in his symptoms.

The following chart gives the correspondences for the above diagnostic indications with their associated Elements.

	Wood	Fire	Earth	Metal	Water
Emotion	Anger	Joy	Sympathy	Grief/Sadness	Fear
Colour	Green	Red	Yellow	White	Blue/Black
Sound	Shout	Laugh	Sing	Weep	Groan
Odour	Rancid	Scorched	Fragrant	Rotten	Putrid
Taste	Sour	Bitter	Sweet	Pungent	Salty
Season	Spring	Summer	Late Summer	Autumn	Winter
Climate	Windy	Hot	Humid/Damp	Dry	Cold
Officials	Liver	Heart	Spleen	Lungs	Kidneys
	Gall-Bladder	Small-Intestine	Stomach	Large-Intestine	Bladder
		Heart-Protector			
		Triple-Burner			

SYMPTOMS

By enquiring about the nature of the symptoms, the practitioner may be able to determine which Officials are causing problems for the patient. If the patient has a firm diagnosis of gall-stones, based on X-rays, then obviously the Gall-Bladder Official must be in some distress. This does not necessarily mean that treatment should be concentrated on this Official. The Gall-Bladder may only be in trouble because another Official is malfunctioning. Only when the symptom is considered along with the pulse, tongue and other diagnostic indications can the practitioner reach a conclusion concerning the origin of the illness.

Symptoms often cannot be attributed to an Official as easily as gall-stones can to the Gall-Bladder. Most can be the result of dysfunction of several of the Officials. Depression, for example, has a totally different quality according to which Officials are responsible. Some people are depressed and anxious, some are excessively melancholic, many are depressed largely because of repressed anger. Headaches and migraines also vary a great deal depending on which Official is responsible. Factors such as the location and type of pain, what brings them on (kinds of food or drink, climatic factors, bright lights, etc), what time of day they are at their worst, the person's constitutional imbalance and many other diagnostic criteria need to be considered before the acupuncturist can begin a course of treatment to cure the condition completely.

An Official may also reveal itself as malfunctioning by 'symptoms' which are not even regarded as such by the patient. The practitioner may realize that the patient is extremely indecisive and this can be a clue to the fact that the Gall-Bladder Official is causing difficulties. Even though the presenting symptoms are physical, after some treatments the patient may well notice a change in his ability to make decisions, as well as in the main complaint. Often he will comment 'I thought that was just the way I was', as he now begins to realize that his indecisiveness was part and parcel of his unique imbalance and that the body and mind are not as separate from each other as he may have previously thought.

24-HOUR CYCLE OF QI

Each meridian has a time of day during which its Qi is at its strongest, and conversely a time when it is at its weakest. This explains why many people are aware that they have times of day when they are at their best and times when they lack vitality. A patient will often describe himself as a 'morning person' or a 'night owl'. This is a good example of a syndrome that is of no interest to the Western-trained doctor but can yield valuable diagnostic clues to an acupuncturist.

Figure 15 shows the time of day when each meridian is at its strongest. These times are based on time according to the sun (that is, the sun being most directly overhead at mid-day) and vary if there are any seasonal changes in the clock, such as during British Summer Time.

I will give the Liver as an example of how one can see the functioning of one of the Officials change according to the time of day. In the early hours of the morning, especially between 1 am and 3 am, this Official is at its strongest. Because of this, a person whose Liver is prone to hyper-function may have trouble getting to sleep around this time of night. This is compounded by the fact that Blood is said to return to the

Liver when the person lies down. It is therefore quite common for someone to feel very sleepy when sitting downstairs but to be unable to sleep when he lies down in bed. One of the main functions of the Liver is to plan and organize, so what often happens is that a person lies awake planning and organizing the next day, unable to 'switch off' his mind. The tendency to be kept awake by the hyper-functioning of the Liver and therefore to become a 'night person' is particularly common amongst drug users who abuse their Livers. Many other people, however, suffer from insomnia caused by this Official, whether on an occasional basis after straining it by eating rich, fatty foods in the evenings or, in more chronic cases, due to a long-term imbalance.

The time of day when this Official is at its weakest is in the early afternoon, especially between 1 pm and 3 pm. It is noticeable that most people's tolerance of alcohol is much

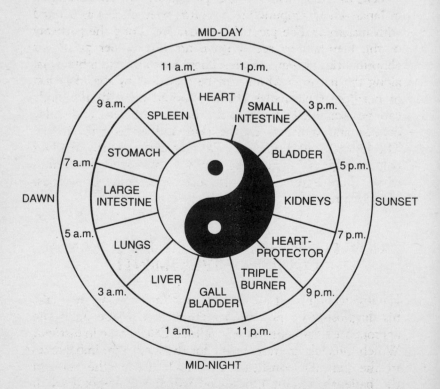

Fig. 15. The 24-hour cycle of Qi

less at lunch-time than it is in the evening. Even a 'heavy' lunch with rich foods in it will often make a person sleepy in the afternoon. This syndrome is most marked in someone whose Liver tends to be weak whereas the person who is kept awake at night will probably have an over-active Liver. By questioning a patient about his best and worst times of day – both in terms of how he feels in himself and also when any physical symptoms come on or are at their worst – the acupuncturist can obtain much useful information about the condition of the Officials.

TOUCH

Touch is another of the major diagnostic techniques used by acupuncturists to discern malfunctioning of the Officials. Touch, as a diagnostic tool, is particularly highly developed in Japan where acupuncture has often been closely associated with massage.[9] The practitioner may feel along the pathway of the meridian to see if there are any tender points or abnormalities of temperature. These may indicate a blockage along the pathway which can be remedied by the insertion of needles at particular points. Various areas of the body can be examined to assess the balance of heat and cold, dryness and moisture in the skin and underlying tissues. The Japanese make great use of a technique which involves palpating the abdomen in various positions to ascertain where there is tenderness or excessive hardness or softness of muscle tone.

HOW DOES THE ACUPUNCTURIST PLAN A COURSE OF TREATMENT?

Having accumulated all the information necessary to make his diagnosis, the practitioner must then decide upon the appropriate treatment strategy. Which Officials are in distress? Which Officials are responsible for the long-term imbalances in the person's constitution? Which are at the root of the patient's current illness and which will respond when the underlying imbalance is treated? Should one treat the underlying imbalance on its own or are there acute symptoms, for example caused by an invasion of Heat, Cold, Wind, Damp or Dryness, which need to be treated first? Are the Officials in excess or deficiency? Would warming the meridian with moxibustion be appropriate?

By combining the diagnostic techniques outlined in this chapter all these questions can be answered.

The acupuncturist will also constantly refer to the diagnostic techniques given here in order to evaluate improvement in the patient. Even if the symptoms are improving, the practitioner will not be satisfied unless he can discern a significant improvement in the pulse, tongue and the other diagnostic indications. For they are the windows through which the acupuncturist can gaze at the balance of the individual's Qi. If these are not responding to treatment, the energetic cause of the person's illness still remains. Symptomatic improvement will only be short-lived. When the patient's symptoms are better, and this is combined with clear evidence of energetic change, then both patient and practitioner can be assured that the treatment has reached to the very core of the illness.

6

What To Expect From An Acupuncture Treatment

WOULD ACUPUNCTURE BE SUITABLE FOR ME?

TRADITIONALLY ACUPUNCTURE HAS been used to treat almost the entire spectrum of illness; physical and psychological, acute and chronic. The following conditions (using Western medical terminology) are amongst the most commonly seen by acupuncturists in the West:

Diseases of the circulatory system

angina, atherosclerosis, chronic heart failure, high blood pressure, palpitations, poor circulation.

Diseases of the respiratory system

asthma, chronic breathlessness, chronic bronchitis, hayfever.

Diseases of the digestive system

colitis, constipation, diarrhoea, irritable bowel syndrome, indigestion, stomach ulcers.

Diseases of the urinary and reproductive systems

cystitis, impotence, incontinence, infertility, irregular periods, morning sickness, pre-menstrual syndrome, prostatitis.

Diseases of the skin

acne, eczema, psoriasis.

87

Neurological and musculo-skeletal diseases

arthritis, back pain, Bell's palsy, epilepsy, headaches, migraines, multiple sclerosis, neuralgia, rheumatism, sciatica, sports injuries, stiff neck, strokes, tinnitus.

Acute infections

bronchitis, common cold, food poisoning, hepatitis, influenza, sinusitis, ear infections.

Mental and emotional syndromes

anxiety, depression, eating disorders, insomnia.

This is not intended to be a definitive list and if you think that your own condition is not covered by any of the above categories you can contact a properly qualified acupuncturist and ask if he thinks acupuncture would be appropriate. Nearly all patients who come for acupuncture in the West have already consulted a Western-trained physician for their condition. If they have not, the acupuncturist may possibly ask them to see their doctor. Acupuncturists do not regard their therapy as inevitably the single most appropriate treatment for each patient. They may sometimes refer a patient to another discipline such as Western medicine, chiropractic or psychotherapy, either as an adjunct to acupuncture or as an alternative.

WHAT IF I AM ALREADY RECEIVING TREATMENT FOR MY CONDITION?

Occasionally it is desirable for the intensive treatment of an acute condition to be completed, for example, a course of antibiotics or chemotherapy administered in a hospital, before beginning acupuncture treatment. Generally speaking, however, it is very rare for any form of treatment to be so incompatible with acupuncture as to make treatment inadvisable. If you are taking prescribed medication for your condition you should normally inform your doctor that you are receiving acupuncture treatment. In many instances it will be possible to reduce or entirely eliminate your need for medication and it is to be hoped that your doctor will be only too happy to be kept in touch and consulted during this process.

WHAT ACTUALLY HAPPENS WHEN I VISIT AN ACUPUNCTURIST?

As in any other system of medicine, on the first visit the practitioner will gather the information necessary to make an accurate diagnosis. If the practitioner takes a holistic approach to the person's illness he will probably allow about one hour and a half for the initial consultation; some practitioners schedule longer, some less. Once the acupuncturist has reached a diagnosis and decided upon the appropriate treatment, he will insert acupuncture needles into various acupuncture points. The number and location will depend on the treatment strategy; the practitioner may use just one or two points in a treatment, sometimes he may prefer to use several points. There are 365 points on the main meridians but there are also many hundred 'extra' points which are sometimes used.

There is usually no apparent correlation between the site of the symptom and the location of the points used. The choice of points is determined by the pathway of the meridians that the acupuncturist has decided lie at the heart of the imbalance. The most commonly used points are located on the limbs, between the elbow and finger-tips and below the knee. Points which lie close to the site of a symptom are used, however, if the acupuncturist diagnoses a localized obstruction in the flow of Qi or Blood. 'Local' points are used most commonly and effectively in the treatment of pain.

The practitioner will manipulate the needles as he inserts them and they may be left in for some minutes or removed almost immediately depending on the effect the practitioner wishes to achieve upon the patient's Qi. The depth of insertion, usually a few millimetres, varies according to the point's location on the body. Unlike an injection with a hypodermic needle or pricking oneself with a sewing needle, acupuncture

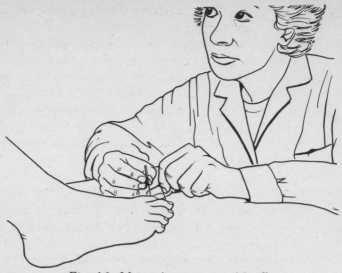

Fig. 16. Using Acupuncture Needles

does not draw any blood owing to the extreme fineness of the needles used.

Will I feel the needles?

Acupuncture needles are so fine that the prick of the needle as it goes through the skin is barely felt. When the needle reaches the required depth and touches the flow of Qi in the meridian, a very remarkable thing happens. 'When the Qi is obtained, it is like a fish that has taken the bait' and 'When the Qi arrives it is like a flock of birds or the breeze in the waving millet' are traditional descriptions of the experience felt simultaneously by the patient and, less strongly, by the practitioner. This is a distinctive sensation which is often described as a dull ache or a tingling sensation and can sometimes be felt along the pathway of the meridian. This sensation is known as 'De Qi' and indicates to both practitioner and patient that the point has been accurately located. The sensation only lasts for a second or two, even if the needles are left in for some time. Many patients comment that having needles was nothing like as bad as they had imagined. As evidence that it is not too disagreeable, it is striking that almost all acupuncturists receive treatment themselves!

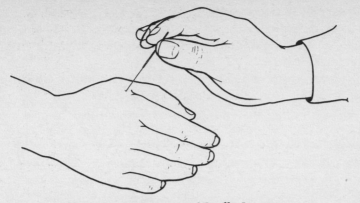

Fig. 17. Acupuncture Needle Insertion

Is there any possibility of infection from the needles?

Properly trained acupuncturists are absolutely meticulous concerning the sterility of their needles and the method of insertion. All acupuncture colleges stress the importance of this aspect of the acupuncturist's practice. *Practitioners either use disposable needles or ensure that their sterilization facilities are impeccable.* In the UK there has been no recorded instance of an infection having been transmitted by acupuncture treatment carried out by a properly trained and qualified practitioner.

Will any other therapies be used?

The acupuncturist may well use other traditional techniques apart from needling. I will give a brief outline of the most commonly used techniques.

Moxibustion

The Chinese term for acupuncture is composed of two ideograms; *Zhen* and *Jiu*. *Zhen* represents 'metal that bites', meaning the needles; *Jiu* represents fire, meaning moxibustion. The two therapies have been practised together for millennia, especially in the cold regions of Northern China, Korea and Japan. The English word is derived from the Japanese '*moe kusa*', which means 'burning herb'.

In the procedure of moxibustion, a small cone of the dried and powdered leaves of the herb Artemesia vulgaris latiflora is placed on the acupuncture point. It is then lit and allowed to smoulder slowly until the patient feels his skin become warm. It is then removed. This is repeated several times on each point. Most patients find that this gives them a pleasant warm sensation.

Moxibustion is used to warm the patient's Qi. This is particularly indicated if the person is deficient in Yang, the aspect of Yin/Yang responsible for warmth. The fact that many people's bodies are always cold to the touch or that they themselves feel the cold excessively is another example of a valuable diagnostic clue in Chinese medicine which (except in one or two specific instances) is of no interest or use to a practitioner of Western medicine. Moxibustion warms the Qi so that not only is it beneficial to the patient's symptoms and general health, but it is also common for patients to comment that they no longer feel the cold so acutely. Moxibustion is used more freely in winter than in summer as this is the time of year when people need warming most and when they are most prone to Cold-related illnesses. Moxibustion is obviously rarely used on patients who are predominantly Yin deficient, who barely feel the cold and tend to find hot weather difficult to deal with.

Moxibustion can also be applied over an area of the body which has become cold; such as a 'frozen' shoulder, the lower back or the lower abdomen (as is commonly found in women suffering from gynaecological problems). There are various methods for warming an area with moxibustion, the most common being a 'moxa stick' which is rather like a large cigar. This is lit and passed backwards and forwards over the skin, just close enough to give a comfortable heat. The acupuncturist will often give a moxa stick to the patient to take home with him so that he can continue the treatment himself on a regular basis. This technique is also extremely effective in the treatment of earache and the early stages of ear infections. The prescription of antibiotics for children's ear infections could be drastically reduced if parents were informed about this method of treatment.

Herbs

Herbs have always played a major part in the health care of the countries of the Orient and in their communities in Western countries. Until recently Chinese herbalism was

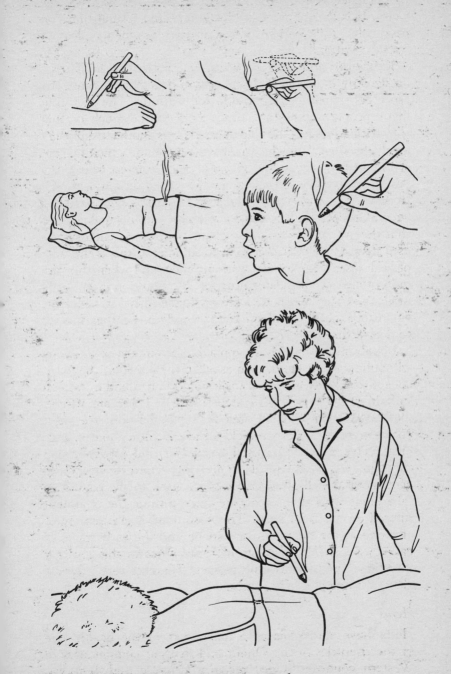

Fig. 18. Moxibustion Techniques

rarely practised by Western acupuncturists as it was very hard to obtain supplies and there were few teachers to pass on their knowledge. Many a tourist, exploring the Chinatown of a large Western city, has been enchanted by the window of a Chinese herbal pharmacy. They have, however, usually been baffled and sometimes ignored if they have tried to purchase anything.

Diagnosis is based upon the same principles as for acupuncture, with more emphasis on Yin/Yang than on the 5 Elements. Many acupuncturists now use Oriental herbs to supplement their acupuncture treatment, often using herbal remedies for a specific symptom, such as to help clear an invasion of an external climatic factor or to build up the patient's Qi or Blood.

Cupping

Cupping is an ancient technique found in many cultures. It was widely used by the Greeks, the Romans and the North American Indians. It is still used in most Mediterranean cultures. There were scenes showing cupping being used in the films Jean de Florette set in France in the 1930s and Zorba the Greek, set in the late 1950s.

Cupping utilizes vacuum suction within glass cups or bamboo jars to disperse localized congestion such as that caused

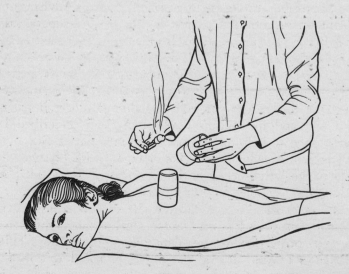

Fig. 19. Cupping

by Wind, Cold or Dampness. A lighted taper is placed in the cup for just a moment in order to create a vacuum. The taper is then withdrawn and the cup is quickly placed upon the skin. The vacuum holds it on and a sucking sensation is felt by the patient. It is not at all unpleasant and is most commonly employed on the back, usually for the treatment of conditions such as the common cold, asthma and back ache. It can also be used in the treatment of joint pains and muscular injury.

Massage

Massage (acupressure) is sometimes used on acupuncture points in situations when it is difficult to use needles or moxibustion. It is not as powerful as using needles but it can still be highly effective. Small children usually have points massaged rather than needled. Sometimes in emergency situations, for example a traffic accident or a sports injury, needles may not be immediately available and the acupuncturist may use massage as first-aid. There are also traditional Oriental methods of massage for musculo-skeletal problems but as yet there are few Westerners trained in these techniques.

Counselling

The Chinese have always placed great emphasis on eradicating, if possible, the cause of a person's illness. Advising the patient on aspects of his lifestyle which the acupuncturist considers are detrimental to his health is regarded as extremely important. This could involve discussion about a more appropriate diet, exercise, the skilful avoidance of excessive stress and how to become less overwhelmed by the various 'internal causes' of illness, the emotions. Traditionally Tai Ji Quan, Qi Gong and meditation have often been prescribed by practitioners to help to harmonize the individual's Qi.

A patient's readiness to make changes in his lifestyle can make or break the success of the treatment. It is considerably harder, for example, for the acupuncturist to improve the condition of the Liver Official if the patient continues to place a strain on it by drinking too much alcohol, repressing his anger or overloading his planning and organizing faculty through overwork. If the patient is prepared to make a commitment to do all he can to reduce certain stresses in his lifestyle, it can enhance his understanding of the fact that he may have a major part to play in the process of returning to, and maintaining, a better state of health.

WILL ACUPUNCTURE HELP ME ONLY IF I BELIEVE IN IT?

Acupuncture is no different from Western medicine in this respect. Seneca, the first century Roman philosopher, said 'It is part of the cure to wish to be cured' and all systems of medicine, even surgery, tend to be more effective if the patient has confidence in the treatment and in the practitioner carrying it out. Some patients, however, seek acupuncture treatment out of desperation and are deeply sceptical about its efficacy. Many of these have been amazed at the results. Believing in acupuncture may be of some help but is definitely not essential.

HOW LONG WILL A COURSE OF TREATMENT LAST?

This will be determined by many factors; whether the illness is chronic or acute, whether the person's constitutional Qi is relatively healthy, how severe the imbalances are, how accurate a diagnosis the acupuncturist has made and whether there are currently any factors in the patient's life which are exacerbating his illness. Treatment may be frequent if the symptoms are acute, but if the illness is chronic it is usual for the patient to come for treatment weekly. This phase continues until the symptoms have significantly improved and the practitioner is assured, through assessment of the pulse, tongue and other criteria, that the underlying Qi imbalances are markedly less severe. Once the patient starts to improve, the frequency of the treatments diminishes. Generally one expects the patient to show some improvement within the first three or four treatments although it may well take longer if the illness is severe or if it has been present for a long time.

When the patient is markedly better, the acupuncturist traditionally sees the patient at the start of each season. It is analogous to going to see a dentist. If you had never been to a dentist until a dental problem developed in adulthood, the dentist would probably have to carry out several treatments in order to restore the teeth and gums to reasonable health. He might advise you how to look after your teeth and gums better in the future. After this the dentist cannot guarantee that no further symptoms will ever develop but will ask you to come in for regular check-ups and will probably be able to forestall any serious trouble in the future. Just as the dentist will often look at your mouth and not do anything, the acupuncturist will question you, take your pulses and may sometimes decide that it is inappropriate to treat you at that time. Another time the dentist may choose to do a small filling rather than wait for a larger hole to develop. Similarly the acupuncturist may decide to intervene with a subtle treatment designed to stop an imbalance becoming more severe. *The acupuncturist's ability to diagnose and treat dysfunction long before symptoms arise, makes acupuncture an extraordinarily effective form of preventive medicine.*

WILL I FEEL DIFFERENT IMMEDIATELY AFTER A TREATMENT?

After treatment it is quite common for the patient to feel energized and vital, but it is probably more common to feel rather relaxed and drowsy. This is because the body needs some time to adjust to the changes that have been brought about by the treatment. The acupuncturist will be able to feel on the pulses that a change has taken place at the time of the treatment, but often the patient will not be aware of any improvement for a day or two. If the patient is suffering from an acute symptom, such as a headache, however, it is common for an improvement to be felt at the time of the treatment. As the *Nei Jing* puts it 'When the evil is a recent guest in the body it does not have a fixed abode and can be expelled'.

CAN ACUPUNCTURE BE USED ON SMALL CHILDREN?

Diagnosis in small children is usually more difficult than in adults and newly-qualified acupuncturists are usually advised not to treat small children. Experienced practitioners, however, frequently treat small children and often find that they respond more readily than adults. Sometimes it is necessary to use massage, moxibustion or other techniques rather than needling. It is a great pleasure for many acupuncturists to treat children as it means that the practitioner can treat the imbalances at an early stage and thereby prevent them becoming more severe and causing symptoms later.

CAN ACUPUNCTURE BE USED ON ANIMALS?

In the East, acupuncture has traditionally been used to treat all manner of animals. Treatment is obviously symptomatic rather than holistic! There is an increasing number of veterinary practitioners in the West who are using acupuncture and in the UK it has received a great deal of publicity after the successful treatment of certain famous race-horses. The long history of the effective use of acupuncture on animals is a powerful argument against the still occasionally encountered view that acupuncture is effective primarily because of the placebo effect.

CAN I HAVE ACUPUNCTURE ANALGESIA FOR A SURGICAL OPERATION?

Although there is a long history of acupuncture being used for the relief of pain, acupuncture analgesia was not used in a surgical operation until 1958 in Shanghai. Its use is now widespread throughout China. It was this modern use of electro-acupuncture that initially attracted the attention of the doctors attending President Nixon during his visit to China in 1972. Prior to this, Western doctors had been inclined to dismiss the results of acupuncture as being due to the placebo effect. That view could not be maintained in the face of patients smiling and talking during major surgery with just a few needles inducing the analgesia. Much research was then carried out to try and discover what physiological effects the acupuncture analgesia was producing. After some time, this concentrated upon the increase in endorphins (morphine-like substances in the brain) and various neurological changes that were discovered to occur during acupuncture analgesia. This work both gave acupuncture analgesia scientific validation and also expanded the knowledge of physiologists concerning how we feel pain and how the sensation of pain can be blocked. It had the tendency, however, of making many doctors think that acupuncture was primarily a method of pain relief rather than a system of medicine traditionally used to treat a broad range of illnesses.

Acupuncture for pain relief has carved out a small niche for itself within Western medicine, treating out-patients in some hospital pain clinics. Results have often not been as good as they could have been, largely due to the lack of adequate training on the part of the doctors involved. Acupuncture analgesia during surgical operations has never become popular in the West and one would probably find it very difficult to find anybody prepared to administer it. There are a number of reasons for this: very few acupuncturists work in hospitals and therefore have had no opportunity to try it out; most Westerners are not as stoical as most Chinese patients and would much rather be unconscious during an operation; it does not produce the muscle relaxation necessary for many operations; it is not as reliable as modern methods of chemical analgesia and few anaesthetists are strongly motivated to explore an unfamiliar technique when their present methods are generally successful.

There are, however, significant advantages to acupuncture analgesia: there are far fewer post-operative complications such as bleeding, nausea and respiratory difficulty; there is no suppression of the immune system as there is with chemical methods of analgesia; the recovery rate is quicker and it is suitable for poor anaesthetic risks, such as the elderly. It will be interesting to see if this cheap and simple method of analgesia ultimately finds a place in either the high-tech hospitals of the West or the more poorly funded hospitals of the Third World.

CAN ACUPUNCTURE BE USED DURING PREGNANCY?

The changes that take place in a person's Qi during pregnancy are so profound that again newly-qualified practitioners are advised not to treat during pregnancy. An experienced practitioner will usually treat during pregnancy only if the expectant mother is decidedly unwell and the diagnosis is relatively straightforward.

CAN ACUPUNCTURE BE USED DURING CHILDBIRTH?

Acupuncture analgesia is occasionally used for the relief of pain during childbirth. However, in order to achieve full pain relief the needles must be connected to an electronic machine and it is therefore necessary for the mother to keep fairly still. Understandably many mothers wish to have a more 'active' birth and in recent times many acupuncturists have been attending births in order to help facilitate the labour in several different ways. For example, acupuncture can be used throughout the labour to significantly lessen the pain when it reaches its crescendoes, to re-start the contractions if they stop for any reason or to draw upon the mother's reserves of energy if she feels that she just cannot go on any longer. Acupuncture, and particularly moxibustion, is also extremely effective immediately after the birth, reducing the likelihood of post-natal depression and restoring the mother's energy and vitality. The judicious use of acupuncture at crucial stages in the labour can transform a woman's experience of childbirth and this could therefore play a crucial role in restoring the confidence of many women to choose to have a natural, rather than a high-tech, childbirth.

CAN ACUPUNCTURE HELP ME GIVE UP TOBACCO, ALCOHOL, DRUGS OR OVER-EATING?

There are usually three reasons why a person finds it difficult to give up a substance which he knows is injurious to his health.

First there is the incontrovertible fact that some substances are chemically addictive for certain people. The most common of these are tobacco, alcohol, certain drugs (prescribed or not) and less seriously, coffee and chocolate. Some people can take or leave a substance such as alcohol – but in others it sets up a chemical dependence that is immensely hard to break.

Acupuncture can be extremely effective at reducing the intensity of the chemical dependence. Much clinical and research work has been carried out on this modern use of acupuncture in different clinics throughout the world, most notably at the Lincoln Hospital, New York. For this purpose acupuncturists predominantly use particular points on the ear, often leaving small studs in position which the person can press if the craving becomes intense. The studs are changed periodically to avoid the possibility of a local infection.

The second reason is the psychological dependency upon the substance. People over-eat, not because there is any chemical dependency, but because it goes a small way towards filling a psychological need. It is often a source of comfort or a small reward, just as a stiff drink is often the 'reward' people give themselves after a hard day's work or after they have finally got the children to bed. The use of these substances to suppress emotions is also common. People often crave the soothing qualities of a cigarette when they are nervous and unsure of themselves in company. The progression from frustration to low-grade irritability, or despondency to alcohol or other drugs is also widespread. [10]

Acupuncture aimed at treating the whole person can also be highly effective in reducing the psychological dependency. It often needs to be supported, however, by an awareness in the individual of his own psychological patterns in relation to the substance, and a degree of will-power so as not to retreat into his habitual modes of behaviour. Finding a less harmful alternative may be helpful if the person continues to feel the need of some 'support' in times of stress.

Thirdly the person may lack the will to suffer some discomfort during the withdrawal phase, and, perhaps more commonly, a commitment to change his lifestyle after giving up. Many heroin addicts, smokers and alcoholics periodically give up their addictions but continue to spend much of their social life with people who still not only maintain their own addictions but also justify them to themselves and others. It is little wonder that many people revert to their addictions when a new supply is only an arm's length away. In extreme cases, such as heroin or alcohol addiction, it is often necessary for the person to enter a hospital, clinic or therapeutic community for a period of time in order to remove himself from temptation. Even in less extreme cases, the practitioner may need to counsel the patient about his lifestyle and encourage him to consider seriously what changes he may need to make in order to minimize the possibility of reverting to his addiction.

CAN ACUPUNCTURE HELP ME LOSE WEIGHT?

If the cause of the excess weight is due to over-eating, acupuncture may well be able to help in the ways outlined in the previous section. Many people, however, put on weight despite eating very little. This may be due to lack of physical exercise but it may also be due to a failure of the metabolism to utilize efficiently the food that it receives. Acupuncture is often effective in making the metabolism more efficient and many patients lose weight during the course of treatment if they are over-weight, just as many patients put on weight if their bodies are too thin.

HOW CAN I FIND A WELL-QUALIFIED TRADITIONAL ACUPUNCTURIST?

There is an old Japanese proverb that says 'Better go without medicine than see an unskilful physician'. On p. 118 is a list of organizations in various countries which distribute registers of acupuncturists who have completed a course of serious study in traditional acupuncture. Any of these organizations will put you in touch with a practitioner close to where you live. These practitioners will be members of appropriate professional organizations, they will be bound by a Code of Ethics, a Code of Practice, and they will hold Professional Indemnity insurance. If you find an acupuncturist by word-of-mouth be sure to enquire about his qualifications and membership of a professional organization.

The practice of acupuncture which takes into account the whole person has always been time-consuming and difficult. It has predominantly been the preserve of an élite, a 'high' form of acupuncture largely unavailable to the masses. The majority of the population have historically relied on the 'folk-medicine' traditions of Chinese medicine, based upon the same principles but practised in a more rudimentary way.

Nearly all practitioners of traditional acupuncture in the West are in private practice and therefore have to charge patients for their services. There would need to be profound changes in the medical and political ideology of the National Health Service in the UK before there could be any possibility of traditional acupuncture being accepted under its auspices. In the UK and other countries, however, increasing numbers of private health insurance companies are happy to meet the cost of acupuncture treatment, partly as a response to consumer pressure and partly because they are increasingly realizing that it can save them substantial sums in hospital bills. Most acupuncturists have no wish to turn away any patient on financial grounds and are prepared to reduce their charges for patients who are genuinely unable to pay the full fee.

It is important to remember that being a Western-trained doctor, physiotherapist, nurse or chiropractor is no qualification for the practice of acupuncture. Some have undergone excellent training but many more have learnt all they know from books and extremely short courses. Be sure to check thoroughly the *acupuncture* qualifications of any practitioner you consult. Furthermore even where the acupuncturist is well-qualified it is still crucial that you find a practitioner with whom you have good rapport and in whom you have full confidence. When you find a suitable practitioner you will have gained access to a system of medicine that is subtle, powerful and effective.

7

Acupuncture: Past, Present And Future

IT IS APPARENT from archaeological evidence that acupuncture has been practised for at least five thousand years. Over this extraordinary length of time the practice of acupuncture has been through a great many changes. During the first two thousand years it is probable that it was relatively unsophisticated: it predominantly relied on stone, bone and bamboo needles and still regarded possession by evil spirits as the sole cause of disease. By approximately 200 BC, however, Chinese physicians, in the earliest texts that have survived, were referring to 'earlier classics' and 'ancient masters' and had already developed the fundamental principles of Chinese medicine that have remained unchanged to this day. This era in the development of Chinese medicine coincided with the dawning of modern civilization throughout the world: the time of Socrates, Plato, Aristotle, Pythagoras, Zoroaster, the Buddha, Confucius and Lao-Tse. The great Classics of Chinese medicine, the *Nei Jing* (c. 200 BC) and the *Nan Jing* (c. AD 100), made no references to magical or religious procedures and they remain essential reading for the student of acupuncture to this day. Since that time many acupuncturists have written books in order to convey their own knowledge and wisdom. Perhaps the most famous of these was Wang WeiYi (around AD 1026) who wrote the *Classic of the Bronze Man*, which contained descriptions of 657 points on the human body. Commissioned by the Emperor, he also supervised the casting of various bronze statues upon which the meridians were engraved and the points located by small holes. The first two statues were placed in the Emperor's palace and the Imperial Academy of Medicine in Beijing and these became the source of the greatest authority for the location of points up until recent times. Before students took their examinations the statues were coated with wax and the interior filled with water. The students had to needle the figure and release streams of fluid from the points in order to pass.

Despite universal acceptance of the fundamental principles, one should not get the impression that the actual practice of acupuncture has ever been standardized throughout the East. It has been predominantly taught from father to son, master to apprentice, and practitioners have always evolved their individual styles. Until recent times, communication throughout China and the East was difficult, hazardous and slow. Each area, each village even, developed its own style and emphasis. For example, acupuncturists in Japan have always favoured the use of moxibustion and very delicate needle techniques whereas in Southern China moxibustion is seldom used and the needling is considerably more brusque!

THE IMPACT OF THE WEST ON CHINESE MEDICINE

The introduction of Western medicine into the countries of the East coincided with the era when, for the first time, the people of these countries were forced to acknowledge the overall technological superiority of other cultures over their own. For example, although there are records of surgery being carried out in China over 1000 years ago, it had almost completely disappeared until the arrival of Christian missionaries in the nineteenth century. The impact on Chinese society was electrifying. It is hard for us to imagine how devastating this realization was to the Chinese, a people who had always been supremely confident that their culture far surpassed any other on Earth and whose word for foreigners literally translates as 'foreign devils'.

There were movements throughout the nineteenth century in all the countries of the East to adopt the technologies and scientific values of the West and in medicine it meant that traditional concepts and practices came under heavy attack. With the fall of the Manchu dynasty in 1911 and the birth of the new republic, the reaction against traditional values and beliefs became even more powerful. In 1914 the Minister of Education declared 'I have decided to abolish Chinese medicine and to use no more Chinese remedies as well'.

Chinese medicine was forced increasingly onto the defensive when Chiang Kai-Shek took power and the 'West is best' era reached its height. Financial support for the teaching of Chinese medicine was completely withdrawn. Nevertheless acupuncture, predominantly in a simple folk-medicine form, continued to be practised extensively throughout the whole of China. The advent of the communist regime in China, however, initiated great changes in the study and practice of Chinese medicine. At first it was dismissed by the leading thinkers as being out of tune with the supposedly 'scientific' principles of Marxism[11] and its teaching and practice were not supported by the government in Beijing. By 1954 it was no longer being described as 'feudal medicine' but as the 'medical legacy of the motherland' and its practice was rapidly incorporated into the Chinese health-care system. Funding was made available for clinics, hospitals and colleges. In 1958 Mao declared Chinese medicine 'a great treasure-house' and he himself frequently used it in order to maintain vitality into his old age. This is also apparently common practice amongst the current political leaders.

The pressing need to provide a system of health care for every member of its enormous population has meant that clear, speedy and direct diagnosis and treatment has largely replaced the complex task of making an individual diagnosis, unique to each sufferer. The practice of acupuncture in China has consequently been simplified and systematized in such a way as to make it possible to use it as a system of mass medicine.

The political climate has meant also that the theories of Chinese medicine have been adjusted in order to be more in keeping with the spirit of the age. The theory of Yin/Yang, always the primary principle of herbalism, has also become pre-eminent in acupuncture. Yin/Yang partly found theoretical favour in the 1950s because, according to Maoist thinking, it is 'a rudimentary dialectic' whereas the 5 Elements, with its greater emphasis on the 'spirit' of each

Element, 'inevitably leads those who utilize it to sink into idealism and metaphysics.' Acupuncture, emphasizing diagnosis and treatment based on the 5 Elements, is therefore more widely practised now in Japan, Korea, Taiwan and the countries of the West than it is in China itself.

There are also many cultural differences in the practice of medicine between the East and West. One of the major differences is in the perception of the nature of psychological symptoms. The Chinese family organization, imbued with Confucian ethics, places great emphasis on self-control and social decorum. This is commonly regarded as the reason for the low incidence of alcoholism, with its tendency to loosen inhibitions. Most people will not admit psychological problems to a non-family member for fear of losing face and of creating difficulties in arranging future marriages, either for themselves or other family members. Western forms of psychotherapy and counselling, when they have been tried, have been notoriously unsuccessful amongst the people of the East. Individuals tend to channel their problems into somatic complaints or, in China, in the extraordinarily high incidence of the diagnosis of neurasthenia.

Neurasthenia, meaning literally nerve-weakness, was a diagnosis frequently given in the West in the late nineteenth and early twentieth century to account for all manner of psychological symptoms such as anxiety, lethargy and melancholia. Treatment varied considerably over the years, ranging from drugs, to a change of air, from exercise to complete lack of exercise, as in the Weir–Mitchell treatment where patients were not allowed even to feed themselves. It fell from favour as a diagnosis as more came to be understood about the functioning of the nervous system, and then depression became the common diagnosis given to people who would formerly have been diagnosed as suffering from neurasthenia.[12] In China, however, doctors still regard it as the second most common illness, only exceeded by upper respiratory disorders. It fits into Chinese cultural values, where lassitude and many other non-specific complaints can be ascribed, without stigma, to the patient's 'nerves'.

The introduction of Chinese medicine to the West has inevitably brought about great changes in the way that it is practised and perceived. Practitioners and patients in the East are steeped in the vocabulary and principles of Chinese medicine in a way that Western patients will never be. Acupuncturists frequently find themselves in the position of having to educate their patients in the concepts of Chinese medicine before they can carry on any meaningful dialogue about the diagnosis or intended treatment.

Both patients and practitioners in the West have been raised, consciously and unconsciously, on the ideas and world-view of the Judaeo-Christian tradition, Aristotelian logic, classical physics, Cartesian dualism, Freudian insights and many other influences totally alien to traditional Chinese ways of thinking. It will be fascinating to see what long-term effects this enormous cultural difference will have upon the practice of Chinese medicine amongst Western Practitioners.

THE IMPACT OF WESTERN MEDICINE UPON CHINESE MEDICINE

Western medicine has certainly posed the greatest conceptual challenge to the principles of Chinese medicine that it has ever had to face. Ted Kaptchuk, a Western doctor and practitioner of Chinese medicine, has written

> no honest Chinese physician can fail to be awed by the achievements of Western medicine, by the ease with which a drug such as streptomycin, or a technique such as open heart surgery, can penetrate to the core of disorders that Chinese medicine finds complex and intractable.

There are few who doubt that Western medicine is superior to Chinese medicine in many cases; particularly those where surgery is effective or where powerful treatment is required in acute situations.

What this has meant is that throughout the East both systems of medicine are practised alongside each other; the patient is free to choose whichever she prefers, often resorting to the other if the first system tried is unsuccessful. Chinese medicine remains immensely popular throughout the East. Hundreds of millions of people have used both systems of medicine and now choose to consult either a Western doctor or a practitioner of Chinese medicine, depending on the situation.

In China they have adopted the policy of the 'three roads'; Western medicine, Chinese medicine and a combination of the two, so-called 'new acupuncture'. This third 'road' has led many Chinese doctors, trained in both systems, to attempt to fit the practice of Chinese medicine into the conceptual framework of Western medicine. There is usually no place for Yin/Yang, the 5 Elements or even the concept of Qi in the 'new acupuncture'. This has led to the quality of the acupuncture being hopelessly compromised as attempts have been made to use it with the symptomatic approach of Western medicine.

RESEARCH INTO ACUPUNCTURE

One of the challenges for acupuncture in modern times has been to prove that it truly is effective. A great deal of research has been carried out in China and Japan but much of it has not satisfied the criteria of the Western scientific method. A major stumbling block has been that the Chinese will not normally use a control group (receiving placebo treatment in 'sham' acupuncture points) in the firm belief that it is unethical to deprive a patient of treatment which experience has shown to be effective. Despite this, in 1979 the World Health Organization completed a thorough investigation into the efficacy of acupuncture and concluded, 'The sheer weight of evidence demands that acupuncture must be taken seriously as a clinical procedure of considerable value'.

Another problem concerning research into acupuncture is that diagnosis and treatment in traditional acupuncture can only be made by integrating a great many variables, such as pulse, tongue, tone of voice, colour of the face, etc. The nature and method of scientific research, however, is to control and eliminate variables. Two patients with an identical diagnosis and treatment strategy in Western medicine will receive in traditional acupuncture a totally different diagnosis and treatment from each other. Much of the Chinese research has been carried out by doctors who conduct research using acupuncture as though as it was primarily a form of symptomatic treatment. *To conduct a research trial which classifies an individual's illness according to a Western classification, and then treats each sufferer with an identical treatment, is in direct conflict with the basic tenets of Chinese medicine.*

Many trials have been carried out using a particular point to treat a specific symptom, using research methodologies designed to test drugs. For example, much research has been carried out on the use of the point 'Neiguan', the point on the inside of the fore-arm that is pressed by travel-sickness bands. There is now considerable evidence of its anti-emetic efficacy after chemotherapy, operations, during pregnancy and when travelling. This research promotes the use of the point to the benefit of a great many people but it gives a totally false impression of the scope and nature of acupuncture.

Even when a compromise is reached between the criteria of the researcher and the acupuncturist, support for research in the West is often not forthcoming. I was a co-author of a small trial carried out in 1986 at the Churchill Hospital, Oxford using acupuncture to treat patients suffering from chronic breathlessness, a particularly intractable symptom. The practitioner treated one group of patients, making individual diagnoses and giving individual treatments over a two-week period. The patients in the other group received exactly the same number of needles, but not in acupuncture points. The patients in the group receiving acupuncture showed significant improvement in terms of their subjective experience of their breathlessness, and in their ability to walk a greater distance than previously over a six minute period. The results of the trial were published in the Lancet (20/12/86) and received a great deal of attention. Subsequent efforts, however, to find funding for a larger study were unsuccessful. In fact the trial fuelled the misgivings of many acupuncturists concerning the value of such research. Most acupuncturists are in private practice, with no access to the facilities or funding necessary to conduct a research trial. Rightly or wrongly, they tend to concentrate on their own practice and prefer to let the extraordinary history of acupuncture speak for itself and to let their patients bear testimony to its efficacy. Each piece of research published in the medical journals seems merely to increase the number of doctors signing up for two-weekend courses in acupuncture.

Apart from researching whether it works, much research

is also being carried out into how it works. Scientists in many countries are attempting to discover what physiological mechanisms are brought into play when acupuncture is administered. Most research has concentrated on acupuncture's analgesic effect; much less on its curative effects. Experiments on animals and people have shown that three main areas are involved: neurological, hormonal and bioelectrical. Although many research experiments have shown that acupuncture is partially mediated through these systems, it is obvious that other mechanisms are also involved. Many researchers in this field think that when more is understood about the electromagnetic properties of the body, it will be this area that will yield the most understanding about the curative effects of acupuncture. It seems that we must await the scientific discoveries of the twenty-first century before enough is known about the efficacy and the mechanisms of acupuncture for it to find a place in the body of accepted scientific knowledge.

IS ACUPUNCTURE A SCIENCE OR AN ART?

The science of acupuncture is based upon detailed observation of how people change when they become ill. Diagnostic signs have been identified, co-ordinated, systematized and tested over millennia, in order to evolve a rational, internally consistent system. Where Chinese medicine differs from Western medicine is that whereas Western medicine has been linear in its development, Chinese medicine has been cumulative. In the West what was previously thought to be true has often been superseded by new scientific discoveries. In the East the theories of Yin/Yang and the 5 Elements have provided insights into the laws of nature that continue to underpin clinical practice. What is astonishing is that at the dawn of its civilization the Chinese physicians discovered truths about the energetic nature of man that have proved empirically successful with billions of patients, and intellectually satisfying to the keenest minds of the East. In using this system of medicine, present-day acupuncturists are these physicians humble and grateful inheritors.

The art of acupuncture depends upon the sensitivity and

intuition of the practitioner. Albert Schweitzer, the medical missionary and theologian, wrote 'It is our duty to remember at all times and anew that medicine is not only a science, but also the art of letting our own individuality interact with the individuality of the patient'. The choice and number of points, the quality of needle technique and the practitioner's ability to make rapport with a person's spirit are crucial factors in determining the success of the treatment. For this reason it is essential that one consults a practitioner who possesses both a thorough grasp of the scientific method of acupuncture and the sensibility to practise it as an art.

THE FUTURE OF CHINESE MEDICINE IN THE WEST

It is to be hoped that the future of Chinese medicine in the West will be one of progressive growth and acceptance as more people have the opportunity to judge its benefits for themselves. The strengths of Chinese medicine complement the weaknesses of Western medicine so elegantly that it is probable that patients will increasingly consult practitioners of both systems in their efforts to find an effective therapy. Neither system possesses all the answers. Far from it. Western medicine has many strengths which are well known to us. Its major weaknesses stem from the impersonal way in which it is frequently practised, its separation of body, mind and spirit and its reliance upon symptomatic treatments to counteract the biochemical consequences of illness. If one's Qi is imbalanced in such a way that some of one's symptoms are at the level of mind and spirit, so that one no longer has a feeling of overall well-being, then Western medicine has very few treatments to offer. Unless the doctor finds some pathological cause, there is only a narrow range of drugs from which to prescribe. These are chiefly the anti-depressants and tranquillizers. These are often effective in reducing the worst of the symptoms but, because of the side-effects, most people who take them feel far from well and are aware that the drugs are merely overlaying the root of the problems. Acupuncture's efficacy in improving a person's feeling of well-being is one of its greatest strengths. As the *Nei Jing* states 'If the body is healthy and the mind suffers, illnesses arise in the meridians. Moxibustion and needles are the proper treatment.'

Westerners are fortunate in being able to receive high-quality Western medicine when it offers the optimum treatment for their condition. Many patients in the West, however, are increasingly searching for a system of preventive medicine which can effectively enhance healthy function. They want to consult a practitioner who possesses the means to assist the natural homoeostatic processes. There are times to 'fight illness' from outside and there are times to use a powerful therapy to strengthen the healthy functioning of the body, mind and spirit in order to cure the illness from within. As Albert Schweitzer wrote, 'Each patient carries his own doctor inside him. They come to us not knowing that truth. We are at our best when we give the doctor who resides within each patient a chance to go to work.'

Chinese medicine's vision of the human being as an integral part of his environment, a microcosm of the macrocosm of nature, strikes a deep chord with many people disenchanted with the materialist viewpoint of Western science and medicine. They are increasingly looking for a system of medicine that acknowledges that the human being is much, much more than just an extraordinarily sophisticated biochemical and mechanical machine. The human being's destiny is to stand 'between Heaven and Earth': to be composed of both spirit and flesh. Traditional acupuncture is based upon this truth and it offers a means to heal the ills of both.

Notes

1. Throughout this book the term 'Chinese medicine' is used to mean the system of medicine which originated in China in antiquity and has formed the theoretical basis of the medical systems which developed in China and its neighbours, such as Japan, Korea, Taiwan, and Vietnam.

2. Throughout this book the term 'Western medicine' is used to mean that system of medicine, sometimes known as Allopathy, which mainly uses drugs and surgery to treat illness.

3. Wherever the terms 'acupuncturist' or 'acupuncture practitioner' appear in this book it is assumed that it refers to somebody who has undertaken a serious and lengthy study of traditional acupuncture.

4. This conceptual leap for the Westerner, unused to the notion of Qi, becomes a smaller step once one considers the implications of some of the discoveries of modern particle physics. Einstein proved that energy and matter, previously thought to be entirely different in nature, are in fact inherently the same. This is summarized by the famous equation $E=mc^2$ deduced from his special theory of relativity. This is why some authorities have translated Qi as 'matter-energy' to try to convey to sceptical Western scientists that the concept of Qi is not as 'unscientific' as it first appears. There is currently much speculation amongst physicists as to whether this sub-atomic realm might reveal a scientific explanation of how the mind and body constantly interact with one another. If so, this will undoubtedly reverse the trend of Western medicine, which is to draw a rigid distinction between *psyche* and *soma*. It has been said that it took 200 years for Western medicine to assimilate the implications of Newtonian physics. It may take 200 years until it develops to the extent that it can incorporate many of the conceptual advances of Einsteinian physics.

5. Two examples of these points are: 1) A point on the breast-bone on a level mid-way between the nipples on a man. (On a woman you will need to assess this spot somewhat by eye.) If the Qi in the person's chest is weak, then this point will often be quite painful if pressed. This was well known to doctors in this country until quite recently and certainly there are few smokers who can press this point without some discomfort.

115

2) Many women, especially those who suffer from a degree of hormonal imbalance associated with their menses, will find that an acupuncture point, situated just below their knee on the inside of their leg, will become painful to touch around the time of their period. Interestingly this point is rarely tender on a man.

6. The *Nei Jing* discussed the circulation of blood in the body over 1700 years before William Harvey's celebrated discovery in 1624.

7. See Chapter 6 for a list of physical complaints commonly treated with acupuncture.

8. Throughout this book when an organ – or further on in the book some other term – is being referred to in the context of Chinese medicine the word will begin with a capital letter.

9. Japanese society in the late nineteenth century was at the height of its 'West is best' phase and in 1895 the practice of acupuncture by practitioners who were not also doctors of Western medicine was banned. There was, however, a long tradition of blind acupuncturists and masseurs in Japan and an exemption was granted for practitioners who were blind. Until the legislation was repealed in 1947 the practice of acupuncture based on traditional theories was carried out almost entirely by the blind and even to-day fifty per cent of Japanese acupuncturists are blind. This has led to the development of styles of acupuncture which use touch to a greater degree than anywhere else in the world.

10. It should always be remembered that however pleasing the effect in the short-term, in the long-term alcohol and drugs further strain the Liver and Gall-Bladder, the Officials most closely associated with a tendency to frustration and irritability. Thus the cycle perpetuates itself – irritability and despondency lead to alcohol and drugs and they, in turn, lead to more irritability and despondency.

11. Marxism, coinciding with the growth of science in the late nineteenth century, was often put forward as a 'scientific', and therefore rational, political theory by its early proponents.

12. The phrases 'nervous breakdown' and 'getting on my nerves' are a legacy from the era of neurasthenia.

Further Reading

Bensoussan, A. *The Vital Meridian*, Churchill Livingstone.
A review of acupuncture research carried out so far.

Eisenberg, D. *Encounters with Qi. Exploring Chinese Medicine*, Jonathan Cape.
An entertaining exploration of Chinese medicine in contemporary China.

Hammer, L. *Dragon Rises, Red Bird Flies*, Crucible Books.
A discussion of Chinese medicine and Western psychology.

Kaptchuk, T. *The Web That Has No Weaver*, Rider Books.
A detailed and intelligent exposition of the concepts and practice of Chinese Medicine. Concentrates on Yin/Yang rather than the 5 Elements.

Lao-Tzu, *Tao Te Ching*,
The great classic of Daoism. Numerous translations: everybody has their own favourite; mine is the Richard Wilhelm edition.

Larre, C., Rochat de la Vallée, E., and Schatz, J., *Survey of Traditional Chinese Medicine*, Institut Ricci, Paris, and Traditional Acupuncture Foundation, Maryland.
A somewhat advanced book, but excellent for conveying the spirit of Chinese medicine.

Macioca, G. *The Foundations of Chinese Medicine*, Churchill Livingstone.
The most clearly written text-book on Chinese medicine.

Unschuld, P. *Medicine in China – A History of Ideas*, University of California Press.
The most comprehensive history of Chinese medicine.

Veith, I. (trans.,) *The Yellow Emperor's Classic of Internal Medicine*, University of California Press.
The only, but poor, translation in print of the first part of the *Nei Jing* (The Su Wen).

Useful Addresses

Address list of professional organizations of traditional acupuncturists.

UK

Council for Acupuncture,
179 Gloucester Place,
London,
NW1 6DX.
Tel: 071–724–5756.

USA

American Association of Acupuncture and Oriental Medicine,
c/o National Acupuncture Headquarters,
1424 16th Street, NW,
Suite 501,
Washington. DC 20036.

Netherlands

NTAV,
Schiedamseweg 92A.,
3025 AG Rotterdam,
Netherlands.
Tel: 476–3858.

NVVA,
Van Persijnstraat 15–17,
Amersvoort,
Netherlands.
Tel: 033–630434.

Australia

Acupuncture Ethics & Standards Organisation,
PO Box 84,
Merrylands,
NSW 2160.
Tel: 681–4836.

New Zealand

NZRA
PO Box 9950,
Wellington 1,
New Zealand.
Tel: 04–8016400.

Index